MW01518855

PRAISE FOR DUCKS IN A ROW

Ducks in a Row is Sue Robins' call to take back patient-centred care from the hospital C-suite and return it to those most affected: patients and their families. This book is less a call to arms than a plea for a more gentle kind of revolution. It's a reckoning that adds music and art and poetry to the clinical sciences. Through great stories and wise asides, Robins makes a compelling case that the time to start the revolution is not when conditions are perfect but right now. You don't have to wait for hospital CEOs to 'get' it. She shows patients and their loved ones how to begin... and in a very readable way.

Brian Goldman, MD, author of The Power of Teamwork:
How We Can All Work Better Together

If Bird's Eye View is the why, then Ducks in a Row is the how-to guide. It is essential reading for anyone who has a passion for health care and dreams of a more human and compassionate health care system, in which simple acts of kindness matter. My business suit is off and I'm heading to the hill. I hope to meet you there.

Emma Poland, Chief Operating Officer, Albury Wodonga Health, Australia

As I read Ducks in a Row, I found myself picturing students in classrooms today as changemakers, leading by example, when it comes to valuing people and their stories. At a time when people are acutely aware of the limits of the health care system Sue invites us to take part in making changes that honour people and the relationships that are at the heart of health care. An expert guide, Sue offers insights about listening, cultivating empathy and inspiring health care 'insiders' to transform the culture to one that centres on belonging and compassion.

Jocelyn Lehman, RN, MScN, Associate Professor,
School of Nursing and Midwifery, Mount Royal University

Sue Robins is the real deal: a pragmatic idealist, a courageous softie, and a singular voice for the power of relationships in healthcare. Ducks in a Row is full of her hard-won wisdom and advice – be the dancing fool and don't be afraid to act with love, but don't give them all of your heart. If you have ever been a patient or cared for one, read Ducks in a Row and imagine how healthcare could be better. If you are a health leader, read and listen. If you aspire to be a patient activist, here is your manifesto.

Robert Maunder, MD, Co-author of Damaged: Childhood Trauma,
Adult Illness, and the Need for a Health Care Revolution

Ducks in a Row is an essential playbook for those of us who want to be a part of transforming healthcare. Sue Robins disrupts the paradigm that a health system must be efficient at all costs and to remind us of the importance of kindness. She brilliantly combines humanity, evidence, and practical tools to upend a system that is provider centred, showing how to shape it into one that is relationship centred. Above all, it is a book grounded in hope that paints a picture of a future state that is within reach and within our power to transform.

Maggie Keresteci, Executive Director, the Canadian
Association for Health Services and Policy Research

Sue's follow up to Bird's Eye View is not only a ducking great read but also a heartfelt guide to putting the care back into health care. Drawing on decades of professional wisdom and lived experience, she offers us a practical roadmap with plenty of warm blankets, stories and humanity. She is the mama duck we need to help us reimagine health care together with patients first and foremost.

Amanda Bolderston, EdD, Radiation Therapist and Researcher, University of Alberta

Sue Robins' new book, like the author, is filled with warmth, humanity, and the kind of wisdom that comes from long experience of being both insider and outsider in healthcare. A golden thread runs through this book: the understanding that healthcare is first and always about people and their stories – and that anyone, and indeed everyone, can help make care better, safer and kinder.

James Munro, CEO Care Opinion

The ugly duckling of the health system is the lack of relationship-centered care. Relationships develop through storytelling, one story at a time. In Ducks in a Row, Sue Robins masterly exposes our mental models and assumptions, demonstrates the need to create safe spaces, and shares how to hold conversations about engagement. Throughout the book, there are very practical suggestions for improvement, or 'ducks'. Acting on even just one improvement adds one duck to your row.... one at a time. This is about OUR health system, about OUR humanity as Canadians. Because each of us connects with OUR healthcare system at some point(s) in time, this book must be actioned.

John(y) Van Aerde, MD, MA, PhD, FRCPC, Executive Medical
Director at the Canadian Society of Physician Leaders

In Sue Robins' newest book, she blends together stories with facts and practical wisdom to teach us how healthcare can truly be better. Sue's book is a call to action: the time to change, to engage with patients fully and humbly, is right now, and not at that point when all our ducks are in a row. We are like the beautifully illustrated little ducklings throughout the book, sometimes brave, sometimes wary, sometimes ready to lead and sometimes waiting for guidance. The strength of these ducklings is not in their uniform willingness to get in line, but rather in their diversity. This book is for hospital administrators, patient engagement leaders and, frankly, anyone who works in healthcare who is willing to pause, listen, and make space for something different.

Yona Lunsky, PhD, C.Psych., Director, Azrieli Adult Neurodevelopmental Centre at the Centre for Addiction and Mental Health

Ducks in a Row: Health Care Reimagined is a timely text that everyone who touches health care must read. A brilliant storyteller, Sue Robins draws on her own experiences in health care to poignantly illustrate the everyday inhumanities experienced by patients. Sue's call to action, a call to focus health care on human relationships is compelling, evidence-based, and beautiful – in equal measure. This book is deeply honest and is an important reminder of the unique and healing power of authentic human connections. I am very grateful to Sue for writing this book now; it is the guidebook we need so we can heal and transform, together.

Doreen Rabi, MD, MSc, FRCPC, Head, Division of Endocrinology & Metabolism, University of Calgary

Sue Robins dares us to dance and be brave enough to put our hands up and start that social movement that begins true health care transformation. Written from words of lived experience and evidence based, this book shines a light on how to be closer to the people using and providing healthcare resources, the importance of the magic of humanities and storytelling in health care. Ducks in a Row explores a reimagination of health care – human beings first. If you walk through the doors of health care in any way, this outstanding book is for you.

Claire Snyman, Author of Two Steps Forward, Health Advocate and Patient Experience Champion

A refreshing account of the very real barriers that patients face in the healthcare system. Reading this, there were so many analogies and points that we had never considered before as clinicians. This book really opened our eyes and we can guarantee it will do the same for you. Sue is a gifted, articulate and inspirational writer who describes the situation from a very raw, personal point of view. The time is now to make positive change. This is a must-read, because all of us at some point in our lives will find ourselves or our loved ones as patients!

Amie Varley, RN, BN, MScN- CP Women's Health and
Sara Fung, RN, BScN, MN, co-hosts, Gritty Nurse Podcast

Ducks in a Row begins with a passionate and thought-provoking look at the current state of health care and the essential need to shift to a focus on humanity for the well-being of patients and providers alike. This timely guide is a how-to woven with a strong and invaluable thread of personal storytelling. Sue Robins' hard-fought wisdom inspires readers, whether receivers or providers of care, to step into the arena of health care transformation and ignite change with practical and proven recommendations to accomplish that goal, one duck at a time.

Karen Klak, Author of Happy Faces Only

How can we reimagine healthcare to change healthcare? Sue tackles the crunch question of whether health care systems built on efficiency can truly address staff and patient well-being. She covers power, hope and ideas, bringing her own humanity and a wealth of expertise to bear. A lucid, compassionate and insightful account.

Miles Sibley, Patient Experience Library, UK

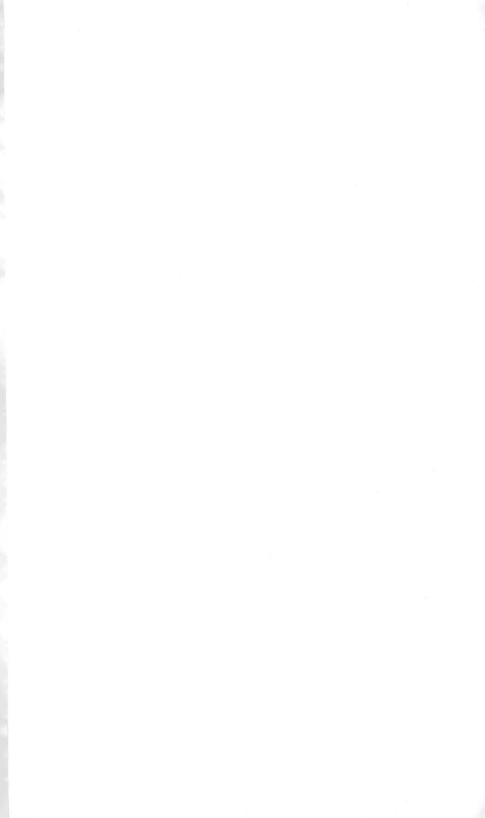

Published by Bird Communications
Vancouver, Canada

First edition.

Publisher's Cataloguing-in-Publication Data

Robins, Sue, author
Ducks in a Row: Health Care Reimagined / Sue Robins.

Includes bibliographical references (pages 209-224).
Preface: A Couch in Melbourne – Introduction: Pragmatism and Idealism – Power to the People – Humanity in Health Care for All – Health Care Reimagined – Conclusion: My Schitt's Creek – Notes – Acknowledgments – About the Author

Robins, Sue–Anecdotes.
Health care reform–Anecdotes.
Health care reform–Canada.
Patient-centered health care–Anecdotes.
Patient-centered health care–Canada.
Children–Hospitals–Administration–Anecdotes.
Children–Hospitals–Canada–Administration.
Hospitals–Administration–Anecdotes.
Hospitals–Canada–Administration.
Canada.

Issued in print and electronic formats.
ISBN 978-1-9991560-4-6 (trade paper)
ISBN 978-1-9991560-5-3 (ebook)

Editorial services from Hambone Publishing and Tara Hogue Harris. Illustrations by Jacqueline Robins. Book cover and interior design layouts by Aaron Mumby Design Inc. Photography by Ryan Walter Wagner. Additional editing and production support from Mike Waddingham.

For more information on bulk orders, or to enquire about bringing the author to your event, please email book@birdcommunications.ca.

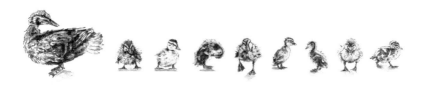

DUCKS
IN A ROW

HEALTH CARE
REIMAGINED

BY SUE ROBINS

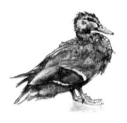

Dedicated to my mentors:

Heather Mattson McCrady, Laurene Black,
Dawn Wrightson, and Catherine Crock.

These women are leaders in advancing humanity in health care.
May we all continue to lift each other up.

TABLE OF CONTENTS

A COUCH IN MELBOURNE

I was perched on a couch in a living room in Australia many thousands of kilometers away from the comfort of my own home. I glimpsed the resident kangaroo in the backyard, reminding me how far away I was from my family.

Jet-lagged and overwhelmed with anxiety, I was nervously practicing my presentation for a health consumers conference the next day. Before me was an attentive audience of two: the couple who had kindly billeted me in their house in Melbourne.

The title of my presentation was *Meaningful Engagement or Tokenism* and it included a photo of a row of ducks. My speaking notes said: "Hospitals, if you are waiting to get all your ducks in a row before you partner with patients, well, that time is never going to happen."

My notes continued: "For patients know that the health care system is deeply flawed; we are acutely aware that we can often end up sicker by having the simple misfortune of being admitted to the hospital."

"As family, we sit beside our loved one's bed on the nursing unit, or in a chair in the waiting room, anxiously awaiting an appointment. We have plenty of time to observe and listen to what transpires around us. We can hear you. We know when the nurses are bickering at the day surgery nursing station, for only a curtain separates us from them. We are unwitting eavesdroppers as you complain in the elevator about 'difficult patients,' or the 'crazy dad' in the coffee line-up; we see you roll your eyes at the reception desk in response to persistent questions from worried patients."

In my speaking notes, I implored, "Don't wait for perfection before you engage patients. Start now".

My hosts, Rod Phillips and Catherine Crock, both physicians in a children's hospital, listened carefully to my rehearsal. Afterwards, Rod paused, delicately choosing his words for feedback, focused on the duck slide.

"Well, hospitals will never actually get their ducks in a row *unless* they start to involve patients and families," he said. A light bulb turned on in my fuzzy head.

With these simple words, my duck analogy was turned upside-down. Rod had nailed the essence of the whole Humanity in Health Care movement.

Your ducks will never be in a row until you partner with the people. Waiting for the little yellow critters to magically align themselves *before* you make space to listen to people and act on what they say is the wrong thing to do.

We must fully reimagine health care in order to change health care. Waiting for the system to change itself is not working. This means tearing down what we have in order to build something new.

Authentic engagement requires involving people as real partners – both at the point of care and in organizations where health system decisions are being made. If health care wants diverse representation with the patients they partner with, they must think beyond the corporate boardroom table. Above all, genuine partnership means treating patients like fellow human beings, not like boxes to be checked off on a to-do list.

People not only have stories to tell; they have experiences to share. Reimagining health care means introducing the humanities into an increasingly science-based world. Art, stories, and humour can bring the humanity back into health care.

Health care will only get better once wisdom is acknowledged, listened to, and incorporated into every level of care and service. Only then will the great revolution in health care begin.

Back in Melbourne, I thanked my audience of two for their comments. My talk was now better because I had allowed myself to be vulnerable and had asked for feedback on my presentation. I scribbled down some new speaking notes, retired to bed early, and presented my talk the next day at the conference centre with my funny Canadian accent to a warm reception from the audience.

We have been waiting too long for the perfect time to reimagine health care based on what really matters. We must reframe from the current corporate model back to caring for each other as human beings. My message in that talk, and in this book, is directed at those who pine for positive change – those who rail against the status quo.

The ducks will never be in a row until there is a re-commitment to *care* in health care. That means understanding different perspectives, adding the humanities and creativity to the mix, encouraging stories, and venturing beyond the hospital walls to go out to the people, to welcome them to participate in decisions which affect them.

Only then will there be a chance of aligning the ducks, or at least encouraging them to travel in the same direction. They need to start waddling towards care and, dare I say, love. This book is a call to personal leadership from anybody who is unhappy with the current state of health care and who wants to reimagine a better world for us all.

PRAGMATISM AND IDEALISM

Pure pragmatism can't imagine a bold future. Pure idealism can't get anything done. It is the delicate blend of both that drives innovation. - Simon Sinek

Ducks in a Row is written for people involved in health care, whether by choice or by fate. Either you have picked health care as a career, or you have been involuntarily immersed in it because you or your loved one is a patient. This includes patients, families, clinicians, students, physicians, and staff. It is a book about us together, not us and them.

This is a follow up to my first book, *Bird's Eye View: Stories of a life lived in health care*. The words here are built upon the foundation laid in *Bird's Eye View*: that all people deserve to be treated with compassion, respect, and dignity.

Ducks in a Row expands on the notion of being in partnership with patients and families beyond the point of care. I use the terms patient and family-centred care interchangeably. Although I've worked mostly in children's hospitals, when I was diagnosed with cancer, I realized the importance of recognizing that adult patients have families too.

This book advocates for a gentler health care system, that incorporates the humanities like art and music. It encourages creating space for everybody to share their stories, both good and bad. It tackles the corporate term 'patient engagement' at an organizational level. The idea of listening to patients – an idea that was once grassroots and led by regular folks – has been hijacked and warped by the executives sitting in the corporate offices. It is now time for health care to be reimagined.

I offer ideas about how to inject humanity into health care, and importantly, I share stories about how to overcome resistance to change. There is always opposition to change, even if it is an objectively positive thing, for human beings crave the status quo.

This book is split into three sections: *Power to the People* examines the problem, the power imbalances inherent in health settings. *Humanity in Health Care for All* is about hope. This section shares stories and best practice for health professionals to engage with patients and families at the point of care or service. *Health Care Reimagined* is the ideas section. It outlines practical tips and stories about creating people-friendly health spaces and engaging folks at the organizational level – on councils, as teachers, as advisors, and in research.

This book is provided as a framework for a new future in health care, but it is not an academic book. It is written to be accessible to all readers. People have devoted their lives to studying topics like patient safety, patient feedback, and the humanities in health care. If you are sparked by an idea, the Notes in the back will help you dig deeper into a topic.

Ducks in a Row is in response to the rise of the patient voice in health care. Patients having a say in their own care has been called many things: patient-centred care, patient engagement, and patient partnership.[1] Whatever you choose to call it, this is surely the slowest revolution on record.

Patients and their families have been speaking up on health

care issues for many years. Their voices have been largely ignored because of a strong patriarchal culture and a great power imbalance between patients and administrators. The rise of the engaged patient movement, Patients Included charters, accreditation, patient safety, and quality improvement initiatives have helped create environments where health professionals and administrators are supposed to be ready to listen to the people.[2] Generally speaking, this has not happened.

This book shares stories about how to listen well to the people. Expanding beyond the concept of patient-centred care, it outlines how to create relationship-centred care. I first learned the term relationship-centred care from Dr. Johny Van Aerde.[3] It means staff and physicians committing to building relationships with patients and families, in a meaningful way, and avoiding tokenism at all costs.

Ducks in a Row is a combination of my own personal wisdom as a woman who experienced breast cancer, the mother of a child with a disability, and my work experience. I've included my reflections on my unpaid and paid work over the past 30 years. I've been a family representative and then a paid family-centred care advisor for three children's hospitals and served as the chair for the Canadian Family Advisory Network, a national family advisory committee. I've been educated at the Institute for Patient and Family Centered Care's Intensive Seminar and have presented at countless health conferences.

These credentials mean nothing. My most important work has occurred in coffee shops, around kitchen tables, and in my car in the parking lot on the phone talking with patients and families. I have been deeply moved by what people have told me. I've had clinicians stop me in the hall or quietly visit me in my office to express their own frustrations with health delivery. Most of all, I've

learned from people like author Heather Plett to hold space for
these conversations, and I've listened carefully to understand.[4]

Many of my examples are from child health. My breast cancer
diagnosis is relatively new and I'm still adjusting to the idea of
being a patient. My son with Down syndrome is now 18 years old
and I've been immersed in pediatric health care for a long time.
When my cancer arrived, lucky me, I was gifted the unique perspective of being both a patient and a caregiver.

This book is for anyone who is tired of incremental change,
often led by consultants with expensive shoes. It is past time to
listen to the regular people who want one common thing: for
every decision, policy, process, and program in health care to be
centred on caring for each other.

 **A note about the little ducks that are scattered throughout
the book. When you see a duck, it points to an idea related
to reimagining health care. You are welcome to steal and
adapt these ideas to your own work. If you don't want to
read the entire book in order, you can simply flip through and
spot the ducks as you plot your own revolution.**

The system is built to say no and turn you away. The machine
does not want new ideas, even if it says it does. It will pat you
on the head and smile in a patronizing way. I want this book and
these little ducks to encourage you to keep going.

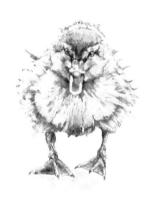

PART 1

POWER TO
THE PEOPLE

Two words sum up this book.

What is the problem with health care? Power.

What is the answer? Love.

It is an act of love to relinquish power. This section tackles the power imbalance in health care. Power is like a pie; there are only so many pieces of it to go around. Folks who have power hang onto those pieces of pie, even hoarding slices, because they are scarce and limited.

This does not only apply to health care executives. From the Department of Health down the organizational chart to booking clerks, people hang onto their power for dear life.

You cannot say you want to partner with patients or encourage shared decision-making unless you are willing to give up some of your power.

As a recent cancer patient, I have witnessed the power mongering firsthand. A card arrives in my mailbox, telling me the date and time to come to my oncology appointment. I am told to arrive early. When I arrive, the receptionist loudly states my personal information for all the waiting room to hear. Suddenly time is important when I am on the clinic's clock. I am not told how long I must wait and therefore I sit in the waiting room seemingly indefinitely. I am called by my first name, or, as I get older, referred to as 'dear.'

The first thing that happens when I am finally called is that I get weighed by a person. Who is this person? She's wearing a name tag, but I can't read it. She doesn't introduce herself or give her title. She holds my chart, full of information about me, but I know nothing about her or even what's on that chart.

I don't want to be weighed but I am not given a choice. I am instructed to take off my clothes and sit in a paper gown until the doctor arrives. The doctor shows up fully dressed. If my husband is with me, she ignores him. She does not chit-chat. She's rushed and seems unhappy to see me. Maybe a patient has died? Am I not an interesting case? I'm trying to summon up empathy for her, but I'm worried about my cancer. She examines me and leaves my gown open, my breasts exposed. I'm trying to listen to her but feel embarrassed to be in such a state. I bring up a concern and she dismisses it with a wave of her hand. She asks if I have questions but leaves before I can formulate an answer. I exit the appointment feeling dejected. Any power I might have had when I walked into the oncology clinic has been methodically taken away from me.

Depersonalizing patients is a way to strip them of power. The system grabs power through their policies and processes, like mailing a rigid appointment time. People grab power by dehumanizing patients, through announcing my personal information in the waiting room, not telling me how long I must wait, and not introducing themselves. The entire interaction with the oncologist left me feeling vulnerable and deflated.

Let us deconstruct how the power balance occurs, both at the point of care and in organizations. To nurture relationship-based care, we must be aware of and acknowledge the power imbalance first.

The key is to start examining personal values and stop blaming the system. The system is made up of people. People drafted the policies and operationalized the processes to create this power discrepancy. We are all the system. The first step is to banish the words 'I blame the system' from your vocabulary.

PEOPLE ARE NOT NUMBERS

A few years ago, I attended a hospital's strategy workshop. There was a lot of lecturing from the podium by people in business suits and presenting of graphs and slides with many bullet points. Not once during the five-hour session was a picture of an actual patient shown on the screen. In fact, patients were not even mentioned, not even once, except in the context of statistics or a data point on a graph.

I could have been at a strategy workshop for a tire factory. I walked out feeling disillusioned about how easily patients were being distilled into faceless numbers. The most demoralizing thing of all was that this was a strategy session for a children's hospital.

I never did see the final strategy document that was written, but I can guarantee that it missed this important point: hospitals exist to care for and serve patients – not themselves. I am shocked every single time I realize that some leaders do not understand this simple concept. Patient, family, and staff stories, shared at all levels of the organization, can remind administrators that hospitals are not corporate businesses. Health care exists to serve the people. Getting carried away with budgets, metrics, and outcomes? Stories can help recentre organizations on the true purpose of their work as caring organizations.

The same thing is happening with the communications about the COVID-19 pandemic from our public health officials. There is much talk about the number of cases, infection rates, and deaths. Those writing the public health communications scripts have forgotten that these numbers represent actual sick people. Real people. Not cases.

Then there are the deaths. These are presented coldly as mortality rates. The people who die every day are followed by the caveat that they were elderly, or they had an underlying health condition. These are shameful footnotes to add to the reports of deaths of human beings – people who were someone's grandma, father, uncle, son, or friend.

I've been treated as a number many times in health care. Before my cancer surgery, I was given a deli counter ticket and called by a number instead of my name.

Why do officials in health care resort to referring to people who are sick as statistics? Often, they hide behind the excuse of patient confidentiality to avoid talking about them as human beings. Are folks afraid that if they know someone's story, or even say their name, they might feel something? This is a sad reflection on the lack of humanity in our health system.

This approach is literally dehumanizing people. People's lives deserve to be valued more than being whittled down into a number at a strategy event.

HEALTH CARE IS NOT A CAR FACTORY

I was working at a big acute care hospital as a staffing coordinator in the late 1980's when the whole Quality Assurance (QA) concept arrived at health care's door. Suddenly everything was about QA this, QA that. I worked with nurses and unit clerks, and we rolled our eyes at all the cute lingo and acronyms that fell out of the administration offices.

The concept of Quality Assurance comes from Toyota, a car manufacturer. It is not about caring. It is about efficiency.

Similarly, many concepts in the Patient Safety Department, such as checklists, are borrowed from the airline industry. This is not about caring. I accept that minimizing errors by using tools like checklists is a good thing, if one doesn't become overly focused on the checklist instead of the relationship with the patient. Patients often describe feeling like a checkbox on a to-do list. As Atul Gawande explains in his book *The Checklist Manifesto*, a focus on tasks is important for patient safety, but I believe only centering on tasks can be a distraction from the core of health care, which should be about caring.[5]

Then came QI (Quality Improvement), TQI (Total Quality Improvement), Kaizen, and Lean. Who thinks up these programs to sell to hospitals? Over the past thirty years these acronyms have all morphed into each other and become one big blob of corporate-speak.

Lean professes to be "a set of operating philosophies and methods that help create a maximum value for patients by reducing waste and waits." Lean also stems from the Toyota management system.[6] I asked a Lean consultant who had been hired by a pediatric rehabilitation children's hospital, "Don't you think this race for efficiency sacrifices empathy?" He insisted that Lean always puts patients at the centre. I said, "Does it really?" and he dismissed me with a wave of his hand.

Just because one says something is patient-centred, it doesn't mean it is true. I don't want the health professionals at the cancer hospital that I frequent taking up their time with wasteful practices like excessive paperwork and administrative documentation. But does this time get reallotted into time with a patient instead? Or is the time saved instead used to cram one more patient into the schedule?

Does pushing patients through the system as fast as you can lessen wait lists? What happens when a patient experiences a safety issue because of this 'fast' health care? Or must return to the hospital because something is missed? Or ends up with medical PTSD (post-traumatic stress disorder) because of the way they are treated?[7] Surely this does not save more time.

"We are allotted 12 minutes with you," a radiation therapist pointedly informed me when I was in treatment for my breast cancer. Twelve minutes to get me on the table, adjust my position, measure me, draw all over my poor breast with a pen, leave the room, radiate me, come back, help me off the table, and then usher me out. Twelve minutes didn't factor in a warm welcome, chit-chat, or space if I suddenly started crying and needed a hug when I was overwhelmed. After all, I was staring at my own mortality while staff progressively burned my cancerous breast with poisonous rays. I was not in a good state.

If I was particularly efficient at getting off the table and leaving the room, what happened to those few minutes of saved time that were sliced out of my radiation appointment? I wanted to donate my time to another patient who needed a minute-long hug.

A lot of people make good money selling these efficiency programs.

A Canadian University advertises a 4-day, online training for Healthcare Lean Six Sigma Green Belt Certification for $2,189. The name of this program is the height of corporate-speak, married with a martial arts metaphor, offered during a global pandemic. The course promises to "Identify root causes of a problem, identify wastes and constraints (bottlenecks), and find and implement solutions."[8]

This approach has drifted out to sea, so far away from the purpose of health care – which is to care for other people – that there's no seeing the shore anymore. Does a health care system built on efficiency lend itself to staff or patient well-being?

In his book *Why We Revolt*, Dr. Victor Montori calls out a health care system that is industrialized, that has failed to notice the patient because of its obsession with volume and efficiency. This is regardless of how the system is funded or delivered. The answer to this, he says, is careful and kind care. This is done by protecting the time that clinicians and patients spend together by making it sacred.[9]

The antidote to the corporatization and industrialization of health care is to make every decision centred on enhancing the relationship between the patient and the people caring for them.

I spoke with a director who works in the public health care sector, who wished to remain anonymous. She shared a glimpse inside the admin suite walls. She explains how corporatization has whittled away at caring.

"Too many health care organization leadership positions today are filled with ambitious executives with varying backgrounds who are 'self-benefit seeking.' Leadership positions earn half a million-dollar salaries, with full benefits that include seven weeks of vacation and plush expense accounts. They are given titles of Chief Executive Officer and are guided by a corporate rule book that would make Warren Buffet blush," she says.

She explains that publicly paid executives comfortably work with business partners like multinational IT providers, pharmaceutical corporations, and diagnostic service providers. The public officials enrich the private sector with large contracts. Communications activities are dominated by a public relations spin. Statistics are massaged to prove any performance goal or population health outcome desired, even if that means suppressing hard facts.

She points out that the practice of patients and families paying for parking was born from a need for a revenue stream that helps to subsidize the 20-year contract negotiated by the parkade operator and its millionaire owner.

"Administrators have boardrooms with comfy chairs, fine-grained hardwood tables, and the latest in technology: smartboards and a wall of video screens. They have so many devices, paid for by taxpayers: the latest phone, laptops, tablets, and home office setups."

She continues the list of extravagances: Executive suites with mountain or ocean views in the nice part of downtown and easy access to the best lunchtime walking trails. Fees in the tens of thousands for head-hunters to attract the top talent. Avocado toast breakfasts, cappuccino bars, and sushi lunch buffets.

A brand-new cancer research tower was built to attract talent and house the newly recruited CEO, while the decrepit cancer centre down the block was left as is for cancer patients to receive their treatment.

She concludes that the days are gone when leadership consisted of dedicated employees with strong clinical backgrounds, who worked to ensure key goals of health care were met by the organization.

Instead, corporatization is killing compassion in health care.

THE UGLY UNDERBELLY

T he COVID-19 pandemic has revealed the ugly underbelly of health care. Pre-2020, internal communications people in hospitals were tasked with keeping health care off the front page of the newspaper. Media outlets were not interested in patient stories. Even if a patient managed to get public attention, the hospital's canned response would be: We can't comment on this for confidentiality reasons. This response was designed to kill off the story.

When COVID hit in 2020, health care workers were lauded as heroes. People stood outside with their neighbours banging pots and pans at 7 pm. This exercise of appreciation faded after a few weeks, despite health care workers continuing to treat more and more patients with COVID. The public enthusiasm to recognize workers waned as exhaustion in hospital environments mounted.

Those working in health care already have a challenging job that is exacerbated during a pandemic. Applauding is not nearly enough.

"About one-third of care aides leave in any given year; many of them take jobs in fast-food restaurants because the pay and the hours are better," says prominent Canadian health journalist André Picard in his book *Neglected No More*.[10]

Health care aides are often not offered full-time positions, so they must piece together several jobs to make a living. Sick pay is not guaranteed and, on top of this, there has been a lack of PPE (personal protective equipment) to go around.

As the pandemic progressed, the shine started to wear off the hero trope. Health professionals began speaking up about their own mental well-being and stories emerged of nurses and doctors who died by suicide. Health care workers were not indestructible heroes after all. They knew that and patients knew that too. There has been much discussion during COVID, including in *The Gritty Nurse* podcast, that the hero narrative is a false one.[11]

Internal communications departments could not stem the tide of patient stories during the pandemic. An Indigenous woman named Joyce Echaquan died in a Quebec Emergency Department because of racism and neglect by the hospital staff. While the hospital pointed to staff shortages contributing to her death ('blame the system'), individuals were caught on video mocking Ms. Echaquan.[12]

Globally, there was a reintroduction of strict visiting policies. Patients had to be dropped off at Emergency Departments alone because they were not allowed to have a support person. People died of COVID by themselves in their hospital beds. Those living in long term care languished for months without any loved ones at their side.

As Kim Crevatin, daughter of a woman who was escorted out of her husband's hospital room for holding his hand, said, "We need to add compassion to the rules."[13]

Patients afraid of being exposed to COVID, or about bothering busy staff, or worried about how they would be treated with non-COVID issues, avoided the Emergency Room even when they needed emergency care. People didn't go for their cancer screenings. The panic about the pandemic was real and had a trickle-down effect that got into every crack of the health system. Pile on increasing deaths due to the opioid health emergency and an impending tsunami of mental health struggles, the cracks are now chasms and the whole foundation of health care, which was precarious at the best of times, was now collapsing at the worst of times.

The question now is what are we going to do about it? Keep wringing our hands and blaming the faceless system?

What if you could do something today? What if it was as easy as having the courage to start dancing on a hill?

DANCING WITH
THE SHIRTLESS GUY

Health care transformation is first a social movement. The *First Follower: Leadership Lessons from the Dancing Guy* video from Derek Sivers explains how social movements begin.[14]

It shows a lone man enthusiastically dancing at a music festival. Sivers says that "a leader needs the guts to stand alone and look ridiculous... this is key – you must be easy to follow." Soon he is joined by what Sivers terms as the first follower. Then others slowly join in. Soon most of the crowd is dancing and it is those who are not dancing who are left out.

The first dancer can be anybody. In my experience, the work to start a Council at a children's hospital began not from the very top, but from a director who believed in family-centred care. She first started dancing alone in meetings, being the only person to put her hand up to question: has anybody asked families about what they think? She did not give up. She kept dancing, connecting with families in the hallways and inviting them for coffee to talk about their ideas.

The director's name was Laurene Black and one of those family members was me. I was a mom from the outside, who initially did not work inside the system, so it was easy for me to join her and start dancing. I invited other families to dance with us, and she invited staff and physicians who were open to the idea of dancing and voila: the change began.

One does not have to be the CEO or a director to start dancing on the hill. Everybody has some influence, no matter how small it may be. Dancing on the hill might be as simple as smiling at patients in the hall and making the time to escort lost people to their destinations. Anybody who works in a hospital can do that. These small acts model the world you want to see and build up over time.

There have been enough consultants in the pre-pandemic times who delivered PowerPoint talks to health executives in boardrooms about change management and health care transformation. I am not interested in rehashing those efforts. I want to talk about how individual people can contribute to change.

Can systems change? First there must be recognition that systems are made up of people. People created the system, so people can dismantle the system too. Change happens one person at a time, and it starts with the guy dancing at the music festival.

I ended up being hired by that progressive director at the children's hospital and was part of a team who built a Family Centred Care Council and led subsequent family-centred care initiatives. Change starts with someone who is brave enough to stick their hand up, to be the first person to get up and dance, even if they are all alone and feel foolish.

I dare you to dance.

LET US GET TO MAYBE

W hen I get a fire in my belly that I cannot extinguish, words guide my revolution. Books are a place to start. To keep up with the modern times, talks are a close second. I've curated my favourite writers and speakers to get you going.

I refuse to call this inspiration. The problem with inspiration is that it is fleeting. Let's move beyond, "Oh, those words made me feel good for a few seconds" to taking wisdom and applying it to our lives. Let these words influence you, not inspire you.

Do not simply read famous authors or listen to well-known people or you will be seeing only a small part of the whole picture. There is a certain amount of privilege that allows one to be published by traditional publishers or to stand on the TED Talk stage. This is a nod to listening to people who do not have a publisher at all, as there are many revolutionaries who have not written a book. Maybe it is your colleague in the next clinic or the patient in front of you. Learning is everywhere if you only open your eyes to it.

Seek local wisdom, and at the same time borrow from seminal books and talks to spark passion.

Audre Lorde was a poet, Black woman, lesbian, and self-described warrior. Her writing about the experience of having breast cancer and telling the truth deeply influenced my first book *Bird's Eye View*.

Her quote opens my book:

And when we speak we are afraid

our words will not be heard
nor welcomed
but when we are silent
we are still afraid
so it is better to speak
– Audre Lorde[15]

If you are happy with the way things are, you do not have to speak up. If you decide to speak up, you will, as Audre Lorde says, be afraid.

The book *Getting to Maybe* is a classic call to action. It was the first book recommended to me when I began working in patient-centred care many years ago. This book is for anyone who has ever thought: This is not okay. I need to do something.[16]

It is dedicated to "ordinary people who want to make connections that create extraordinary outcomes." It is a profound book about social innovation to create social change. *Getting to Maybe* is not specific to health care, but one of health care's greatest challenges is to read stories from other sectors and apply the learnings. Health care often thinks it is special and too complex. Every sector thinks it is special and too complex and we fail when we don't learn from one another.

Who looked at the lessons from the efficiencies in the Toyota car factory and thought: 'Why don't we apply this to health care?' [17]

If a car factory model can influence health care, why can't health care learn from a book about social change? The key is to learn from thinkers who describe the world you want to see. The world I want to see is not rooted in efficiency. It is rooted in humanity.

Getting to Maybe shares stories about social innovators, like a furniture maker in Bangladesh, the PLAN Organization that creates a good life for people with disabilities, and early HIV/AIDS activists. It is a book that explains how to lay a foundation for a movement.

Other thinkers in this realm include Margaret Wheatley, who says, "There is no power greater than a community discovering what it cares about."[18]

Turning to One Another: Simple Conversations to Restore Hope to the Future is a book less about systems and more about personal growth. While it is important to understand system-thinking, the answer does not lie out there in the system. The answer is inside our hearts and begins with the questions we ask each other.

"I believe we can change the world if we start listening to one another again," Wheatley says. I often quote these words. The system is only interested in maintaining the status quo. We will build the world we want to see only by first listening to each other.

Looking to expand your mind? Look beyond health care. If health care really is about humanity, seek writing that examines the experience of being human.

Richard Wagamese was an Ojibwe author and journalist.

> *"Words are less important, less effective than feeling. When you sit in perfect silence with someone, you truly know how to communicate."*

This meditation is from Wagamese's book *Embers: One Ojibway's Meditations.*[19]

Poet David Whyte also writes about having courageous conversations, saying that the courageous conversation is the one you don't want to have.[20]

Reading books is a way to be immersed in other ideas, but videos are easy to access and quicker to consume than books.

 I helped set up a monthly TED Talk session for hospital staff, where a TED Talk was screened, followed by a facilitated discussion. The video did not

have to be specifically about health care, so long as the lessons from it could be applied to health care settings. What if staff other than clinicians were given time to attend a video session? And what if patients and families were invited too?

TED Talks have influenced my thinking about change. A good example is Andrew Solomon's *Love No Matter What*, where he eloquently shares his story about being a gay man and the importance of unconditional love.[21]

I preach about looking beyond health care for wisdom but have my own biases about learning from business. Too often the talk devolves into corporate-speak or marketing because, big surprise, the capitalists are trying to sell you something.

I make an exception for Simon Sinek. His *How Great Leaders Inspire Action* TED Talk is a powerful one if you can put aside the fact that he's speaking about selling computers. What he's really asking his audience to do is to move beyond 'what' you are doing and even 'how' you are doing it – to your 'why.' Your 'why' lives inside of you. I use his talk to help folks dig deeper to uncover their own whys, to find their passion for health care.[22]

If you don't know the work of social worker and researcher Brené Brown, a good place to start is her first TEDx Talk, called *The Power of Vulnerability*. If you already know her work, watch it again. Good leaders are vulnerable. Bad leaders are not.[23]

If you only have 4 minutes and 23 seconds, Cleveland Clinic has a classic video about empathy. Its message is if you want to make all your decisions based on empathy suddenly you will be the change you want to see.[24]

Looking to start a movement? Read books. Watch videos. Get your 'why' in order. Gather people together in coffee shops and around kitchen tables to have conversations about hard questions.

Be clear about why you are doing what you are doing, because that's where the heart of a movement really resides. Be brave enough to stand in your own truth, to speak up, to start dancing, even if you don't have a fancy title or feel your realm of influence isn't big enough.

It starts with one person. And that person is you.

ROOTED
IN LOVE

When I launched my first book at the Gathering of Kindness in Australia, with my friend from the couch in Melbourne, Dr. Catherine Crock, I realized that *Bird's Eye View* is part of a movement. While the Gathering of Kindness was born from the patient-centred care movement in Australia, it evolved into events that "nurture and instill a culture of kindness throughout the healthcare system," and began to shine a spotlight on staff well-being.[25]

This is not just about humanity for patients. It is about humanity for everybody in health care – patients, families, staff, and clinicians. I wrote:

> *"Every single staff member is paid to care for patients,*
> *whether directly or indirectly. This includes the*
> *tradesmen who work in the physical plant, the clerks*
> *in health records, and the staff in food services."*[26]

Staff and patient well-being are issues no matter what country you are in or how the health system is funded. The problems are the same in Australia as they are in Canada, the UK, and the USA. This is not only a funding or a system problem. This is a human problem.

The main trouble is that efficiency has trumped empathy. How I pine for the return of the old-fashioned notion of bedside manner. Kindness could be baked in the system, from how health care is funded; to recruitment of health faculty students; to the hiring of staff and performance reviews. Imagine a health care world that valued listening, tender words and hugs.

There are pockets in health care that lean towards this gentle care, like family practice, pediatrics and palliative care, and other specialty areas could learn from them.

The pressure to push patients through the system as quickly as possible is literally killing both patients and clinicians. If health care is now a car factory, the problem is that patients are not car parts and clinicians are not factory workers. Both patients and staff are harmed by this model. Morale is at an all-time low and patient safety is in jeopardy.

The news flash that we are all in this health care mess together is a novel one. It is patients, families, staff, and clinicians who can band together to demand that we put the care back into health care. Do not look at physician well-being and patient well-being in silos. We are all intertwined.

The key is to reignite passion in health care, to help the professionals find meaning in their work again. If we teach our health faculty students and new staff well, to honour storytelling, to embrace the humanities in order to understand different perspectives, there is hope to turn this ship around. The health care revolution should be a social movement that is rooted in love.

One of my favourite memories in Australia was at a hospital cafeteria. I presented at a pop-up book talk at lunch time in a small rural hospital. The cafeteria was packed with patients, families, and staff. It was a bit disconcerting to speak to people while they were busy eating their meals, but I had a rapt crowd of about a dozen people listening to me as I read two chapters from my book. At the end, I asked: Do you have any examples of kindness you've experienced that you'd like to share?

An elderly gentleman got up and walked over to the podium. I handed him my microphone.

"I want to thank all the staff who have been so kind to us and who helped my wife since she's been sick," he said, tears welling up in his eyes. He paused, unable to go on.

I asked him if I could give him a hug and he said yes, and so I did. Afterwards I sat and chatted with his wife and him. It was a profound and moving experience. It reminded me of the power of allowing patients and families space to share their stories and how crucial it is for us to listen – to deeply listen to understand.

Here's what I proposed in Australia: More warm blankets. More gentle touch. More smiles in the hospital corridors. More healing environments. More chit-chat. More hugs. More reverence for stories and the lived experience. More art. More music. More book clubs. More eye contact. More discussions about TED Talks and other videos. More reflective practice. More rewards for kindness. More pausing before knocking on patient doors. More reaching out to the people (all the people, not just people like you). More love for yourself so that you can love and care for others.

We must focus on the good stuff to stamp out the bad. We must also be honest about our experiences. We can do that through telling our authentic stories and finding champions who will listen.

RELATIONSHIP CENTRED CARE

Hospital websites loudly proclaim they are patient-centred without any evidence to prove these boasts. You can't announce that you are patient-centred until patients say that you are.

Patient-centred care has become jargon, hijacked by the corporate office. Patient-centredness also rubs up against staff well-being. After I presented to a group of pediatric residents, one of the audience members gave this feedback: "You are talking about what you want us to do for you? What about us? We work really hard."

The phrase patient-centred can make staff wince. It has been misconstrued as being all about me, me, me the patient, with no regard for the staff.

A mom once taught me that all relationships are based on this formula: see you, know you, like you, trust you. Often patients only see their nurses and doctors. Without knowing them and maybe liking them, there is no trusting them.

Health care is built on relationships between patients and professionals. You cannot have one without the other. Sadly, often the relationships are not mutual. Patients cannot have a relationship with a person they do not know or trust. If health care folks hide behind professionalism and do not let patients know them, it becomes difficult to trust them.

Power comes into play here. To have a healthy relationship, staff cannot hold all the power. I'll say it again, power is finite, like the pieces of a pie. People must give up some of their power in order to give it to patients – through tactics like information sharing; treating people with respect and dignity; and shared decision-making. These things help form an authentic relationship.

Patients are in many relationships with people who work in health care: booking clerks, cafeteria workers, therapists, nurses, and physicians. Everybody who works in health care should be considered a health professional. Their relationships with patients should be valued and nurtured too.

What if we reframe patient-centred care to build supports around relationship-centred care instead?

"...the context of relationship-centred care, where neither the clinician nor the patient – but the relationship as a whole – is the focus," says Dr. Johny Van Aerde. He is a neonatologist and physician leader who has written about relationship-centred care. He ties the notion of relationship-centred care to the patient experience.

"Although institutions talk a lot about the importance of empathy in delivering good care, there was actually little knowledge of what a patient experiences as he or she navigates the health care system," he continues.[27]

The adage of 'what counts is counted' applies here. I talk about patient feedback later in the book, but I'll leave you with this: How can health care hope to root itself in caring if we don't even ask the people involved if they feel cared for? How do we create environments where people care about each other?

It starts with creating safe spaces for people to be honest. It is as simple and as complicated as that.

DEMOCRACY WAS BORN

Democracy was born
When we boiled the kettle
And laid a clean sheet
On the kitchen table.

Democracy was born
In the needle exchange
With two men, punched and bloody
There democracy was born
When the young woman, the nurturer,
Took them out for a walk
Around the block of the shelter
For a bit of fresh air.

Democracy was born
In a conference hotel room
Sitting on a bed tipping a bottle of red wine
While three moms schemed advocacy efforts.

Democracy is never born
At the polling station
Around the boardroom table
At the bureaucrat's office
Or in the hallowed chambers.

Instead, it lives out loud.
In coffee shops
While breaking bread

On the steps of the legislature
And in the mean streets.
All the new ideas are babies born
Around the kitchen table.

DON'T GIVE THEM ALL OF YOUR HEART

There are lessons in the leaving. I hold insights into the good and bad of an organization when I leave. It's a shame there are not more exit interviews when one departs because there is wisdom there.

Passionate, committed people are eaten up and spit out by hospitals. This happens with staff all the time, but it also occurs with patient representatives who venture into the boardrooms of an organization. The only way to get to what's right is to first talk about what's wrong.

My best wisdom about patient engagement came from Donna, a mom of two and family advocate. It was 2008, and I was sent as a volunteer to an Institute for Patient and Family Centered Care Intensive Seminar as part of a team with a manager, social worker, and another family member. [28]

This was my first time getting 'deep' with staff – spending time with them as opposed to merely sitting across from them at a council meeting.

The teamwork was a disaster. Naïve me thought the hospital staff was interested in my input. They were not.

After one disheartening meeting, I started sobbing in the hotel elevator on the way back to my room. The elevator doors opened, and Donna walked in.

She gave me a hug and invited me to her room. I sat on her bed and continued to cry, blurting out my sad stories of exclusion that had occurred over the past two days. I felt like a fool for having trusted them, for thinking that the staff wanted to partner with families.

'You do this work because you believe deeply in it,' Donna said. I nodded. 'Listen carefully. Never, ever give them your whole heart,' she continued, sharing the most important wisdom I've learned over the past two decades.

I had allowed them to take my heart, and I promised myself not to make the same mistake again. I had to be whole-hearted in my work, but I vowed to keep a little bit for me.

Ah, but the mind is forgetful. It is like falling in love again after you've been heartbroken. Memories fade. Another opportunity came up for a paid position and I accepted that, full of hope and vigour. That, too, came to an end, after four years of important family-centred care work.

I was consulting for a hospital at a senior level. I thought I had a strong relationship based on trust with the new leader. I happened to have day surgery and was recovering at home on my couch when I received some terrible news.

The hospital was planning on firing the coordinator of my son's medical clinic. This would in effect shut down the coordinated care clinic, and children with Down syndrome would no longer have specialized medical services in our health region. Families who were already engaged with the hospital on an organizational level were not consulted or even informed that their child's clinic was going to be shut down.

There it was again: a hard decision needed to be made, and patients and families were left out. That sting of betrayal, and the need to advocate for my son's community, put me in a direct conflict of interest with my hospital position. I left a message on the senior director's voice mail and tearfully constructed my resignation letter. The hospital's values were no longer in alignment with my own, and the associated moral distress was too much to bear.

This was a clash against the strong culture of health care, which today grows more and more corporate by the moment. So odd to treat health care as a business when in fact its core purpose is to care for people and to heal their suffering.

I think of the extraordinary administrators who I know, and what personal qualities make them exceptional. Dawn Wrightson is the (now retired) leader who first hired me. She was a strong believer in listening to families. In fact, she welcomed families into the corporate office, made them tea, offered them chocolates, and listened to their stories. Her nursing heart had not been extinguished over the years of committee meetings, and it still was beating strong.

Laurene Black is another mentor who had a deep understanding of the complex world of families. She was a true rebel, counseling me to keep my head down and keep going when things got tough, but also advising when it was time to throw in the towel, when your own personal values are not congruent with the organization's values. I remember sitting in a food court with her when she explained this to me: you aren't in alignment with the hospital anymore, she said. Either they changed, or you changed, but it is time to say good-bye. Such a profound statement relieved me of my struggle and guilt and set the stage for my eventual exits.

This is not to say that good work cannot be done in the meantime. Hospitals are entrenched with their culture, often in unconscious ways. They aren't even aware how pervasive it is, and only outsiders can recognize this. The problem is that they don't want outsiders to realize it. They think they have all their ducks in a row.

I left my final position at a hospital after 18 months of service.

I pounded out my letter of resignation in my condo parkade, my laptop jammed in between the steering wheel and me, my eyes filling again with those damn tears. At least I could express gratitude in my leaving:

> *... it has been an honour to have been invited to catch a glimpse into the complicated, beautiful lives of families who are served by the hospital. May they continue to find the strength to use their voices and to share their stories to make the world of health care a better place.*

This workplace was not family-friendly enough, I was undervalued for the work I do, and my position teetered on tokenism. By tokenism I mean I was in a figurehead position, with no real authority or power. It looked good to have me there on paper, and nothing more.

The last conversation I had with the administrator was horrible. She was annoyed I had been on a leave with my son, annoyed people kept asking when I would come back, and annoyed that I hadn't been there to remind her to invite a family to be involved on an interview panel. I had become an inconvenience, not an asset, and she brushed me away like a buzzing fly.

I asked if I could go on contract, with a livable rate and flexible hours, and her lips pursed even further. Her only concern was to fill my staff position – when could I get my letter of resignation in? When could she post and interview for the position? I realized with a start that I had only been a warm body. It did not matter who I was, what ideas I brought with me, how deeply I felt about this work, or how many things I had delivered in a part-time position.

The job had to be filled by someone, anyone. They could have stuffed a scarecrow and put a sign around its neck that said, 'family rep' and plopped it in a chair around the boardroom table, and that would have been enough. This was tokenism at its core, and I had allowed myself to be tricked again. I had given them my whole heart, thinking that only working three days a week would protect me. It had not.

I walked away with nary a word of recognition from my manager and tried not to let the door hit me in the ass on the way out.

ALIGNING STARS: THE ROLE OF SENIOR LEADERSHIP

I am encouraging you to take action today, no matter your title, or lack of title. Go out to the people. Make space for feedback. Lean on the humanities like the arts, music, and stories.

It does help to have senior leadership on the same page, but you don't have to wait for them to catch up with you. You can start now without permission.

I've tended to the patient, family, and staff relationships in one hospital that had the highest executive support, Dawn Wrightson, who modelled relationship-centred care in her heart and in her actions.

For another children's hospital leader, the concept of compassion in health care was tokenistic. It looked good to hire me into a family engagement position role. I was fortunate that I was given the autonomy to work away at outreach and storytelling, as long as I made the leader look good. When I started asking questions about peer support and the complaint process, my shine started to wear off.

Guess which hospital still embraces the concept of humanity in health care? The first one. Me chipping away at change all alone, even as I amassed a gradual team of supporters at the second hospital, did not create a sustainable difference. When I left, most of the work left with me. This felt like failure at the time, but in retrospect, I've since realized that even opening up conversations about what family-centred care means is a success.

The first hospital experience began with a question. When given the chance, I would ask the CEO, 'When are you going to start a family council?' persistently and with a smile.

I finagled funding to attend a health conference in Montreal. Two moms and I banded together to lobby for a council. We sat on a hotel room bed with a bottle of wine and planned how we would politely approach the leader. This was a hospital where all three of our kids received services.

We ran into the CEO in the corridor. 'Hi!' we said cheerily, chit chatting a bit. 'Is there a chance at next year's conference we could introduce the new Council?' we asked nicely. The CEO was receptive, 'Yes, we are working on it,' she said. We walked away satisfied that the concept was on her radar.

Note: The real work at conferences goes on in the hallways, not in the meeting rooms.

Change is about planting seeds. Director Laurene Black also happened to have a loved one with Down syndrome, like me. We bonded over this connection and she asked me for coffee a few months later. When you are planting seeds, you need patience too. Things take time to grow.

At coffee, we talked about the concept of a council. I didn't hear from her for a few weeks and then there was a sudden email about me attending an executive meeting in the CEO's office. Hesitantly, I agreed. I had no idea how to prepare so I conferred with my fellow moms to clarify what it was we were asking for. We had vision for about a million things we wanted to change at the hospital, all of which would improve the family and patient experience. But we settled on asking for one thing: a family council to be formed.

I was in the midst of my tenure chairing a national committee of family councils. This allowed me an inside peek into the councils at other children's hospitals. I was not above using comparison to make my point. If other hospitals had councils, why didn't we? This seemed like a fair question.

The day of the meeting with the executive, I stood in front of my closet, fretting about what to wear. Should I dress as a mom or one of them? Hospital executives wore business suits. I pulled out a conservative jacket, skirt, and blouse from my old working days.

I arrived at the corporate offices, sweating and nervous. I had no idea how to prepare, so I just showed up with my fine self and a pitch I had created.

I was directed to sit in a chair by the secretary until I was summoned in. Laurene came out to fetch me. I walked into the CEO's office. There were six high-powered women sitting around the small meeting table. They shuffled about to make room for me.

They looked at me expectantly. I dove into my pitch about starting a council, smiling, and making eye contact despite my nerves. I could see my ally nod out of the corner of my eye. That settled me down.

'Let's talk about this!' I said, a layperson who had not stepped foot in a meeting room for many years. The questions came fast and furious.

'But we've had a council before and it didn't work.'

'If I want feedback from families, I can ask them in the waiting room.'

'The council won't have diversity.'

I smiled again and nodded. It was valuable to hear the perceived barriers directly from the mouths of the senior leaders. I addressed each of their concerns, one by one, blissfully naïve as to the politics in the room.

'It is natural for councils to end – they have a life cycle,' I responded. 'Maybe it is time to try it again!'

'Families in waiting rooms will indeed give you important point-in-time feedback. A council will offer a different kind of feedback – more reflective ideas. This input will be from families who aren't in the middle of a crisis.'

'It is true that councils struggle with diversity. We have to start with what we have and extend out to families from there.'

I did not know that this would be one of the most important meetings of my life. We finished up. I felt wrung out. Everybody was respectful to me, but it was clear there were many concerns. Laurene escorted me to the elevator.

I was surprised what she said next. 'I'll get back to you about a contract,' she said. 'You've put too much unpaid time into this – it is time you are paid.' This was the beginning of my career in patient and family-centred care.

I learned afterwards that my contract as a Family Centred Care Consultant was a result of luck and timing. There had been an executive higher up who was opposed to the idea, but she got promoted and floated out of the way on the organizational chart.

This family-centred care work reconnected senior leaders with their original calling in health care – to care for and serve patients and families. The friendly director had been persistently putting her hand up in meetings for months, asking: 'What would patients and families think?' setting the stage for the council. The stars all aligned because the senior leaders were aligned.

Leadership support is rare. The lobby effort needed to start this Council was real. The timing was right, but it was the persistence of staff and families that really paid off.

Do not give up. Find allies. Keep going.

SHED YOUR PARKA AND TITLES AT THE DOOR

T he children's hospital council had its first meeting in 2009. The holidays were approaching soon after, so we decided to have a holiday party. Hosting a party with this newly formed group of people seemed like a natural thing to do.

It was wholly unofficial, but in cahoots with Heather Mattson McCrady, the Family Centred Care Manager, we went ahead and did it. In the early days, we embraced a 'just do it and apologize later' philosophy. We were pioneers in a new land.

We had no budget and we couldn't serve alcohol in a hospital setting (of course), so my husband and I decided to host a party at our house.

We sent out invitations to the entire Council – senior leadership, family reps, physicians, clinicians – stressing that this was a family party – partners and kids were welcomed. We made it a potluck to cut down on expenses and we had a jar at the door for folks to donate to our booze fund. Heather and I wrote out personalized holiday cards for everyone. I bought sequinned Santa hats from the dollar store for all the kids. I don't know how much all this cost. There was no funding and it didn't matter.

As is typical for a December evening on the prairies in Canada, it had snowed, it was very cold, and the roads were icy and awful. But our doorbell kept ringing and boots and parkas piled up in our entrance as more and more guests arrived.

Here's what I remember: Serving cocktails on a silver platter at the front door. Children running wild through our house: kids jumping on beds, kids running up and down the stairs, kids pulling out all my son's toys (Note: this was all awesome).

The hospital's leader, Dawn Wrightson, was there – her newly-retired husband had cooked an amazing dish for the potluck while she was at work and he had braved the roads to meet up with her at our place. Another senior director came with her two children and husband. Her kids were playing with our kids, the patients – who were a diverse lot, a collection of children with disabilities and medical conditions. Seeing them all zooming around our house – at varying speeds, with various mobility issues – it was all as it should be.

My husband standing in our kitchen, deep in conversation with a dad whose child had died at the hospital the year before. Me, checking on kids downstairs, standing in the doorway of the bathroom, talking to a PICU intensivist while his young daughters ran amuck around us. A neonatologist popped by on his way from his martial arts class, leaning against the wall in the hallway chatting with a mom. It was a houseful of people connecting with people as human beings.

My husband and I hosted this party like every other party we had ever had at our house. Our formula was a bounty of food, fancy cocktails, blaring music, and an open door. For whatever reason, people showed up. I understand now how important simply showing up is. The people who came to that party were providing evidence of their early commitment to the family-centred care cause. For the staff, this was an unpaid, after-hours affair. For the families, this was the end of a long day. But they still showed up. I believe this evening was a tipping point. It was the beginning of a culture change at the hospital.

There were holiday parties like this for three years. The amount of people involved in family-centred care at the hospital expanded and outgrew a house party. The celebrations switched to summer barbecues at parks instead, which was a natural progression of growth.

But those early holiday parties were special. They were intimate and inclusive affairs. There was a complete shedding of roles those evenings. Titles were taken off at the front door, along with the parkas and boots. There was a relaxing of tightly held positions with a cocktail or two. Meeting everybody's partners and kids felt important. By the end of that first dark December evening, we were no longer professionals or families; we were colleagues and blossoming friends.

 If you are reading this and thinking that there's no way a house party with your hospital staff and patients and families would ever happen, here's my challenge to you. If you really want to partner with the people you serve, you need to see them – and your staff – as people first. It is your job to remove all the barriers to create an environment where you would be able to host a party at your house. If this seems impossible, you have to take away the preconceived rigid notion of what it means to be a professional, ignore the policies and procedures forbidding socializing, and fund the damn party out of your own pocket if you must.

This is not a movement created around a boardroom table. Providing opportunities to lose your title and connect as human beings is the only way you can actually seal this deal. Celebrating together – breaking bread, getting to know each other, toasting to the season – is a great way to start.

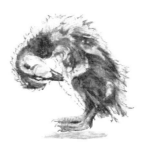

PART 2

HUMANITY IN HEALTH CARE FOR ALL

ndividual champions can make a difference, today, without any permission from their managers and without needing to change the whole system.

There is good work being done. If you are reading this book, you are one of the champions. Pause to think about the good you've done today to advance humanity in health care. This isn't about the big stuff – launching an initiative, finishing a project – it is about the million little things that create a strong culture. And it starts with a smile in the hall.

This section is about valuing people, not dehumanizing them into heroes or diagnoses. It is about us together, and how the well-being of patients and staff are forever intertwined.

In this section I talk about love: love for patients, love for staff, love for oneself. Nobody describes this better than family physician Dr. Kirsten Meisinger in her essay "Love, the Word that Medicine Fears":

> *"...once you start openly loving patients – once you open yourself – you become more effective, not less. My patients know I love them. I remind them when they are getting chemo. I call them if I have been wondering how they are doing, or I know that I can if I need to. And in return they help me. They try really, really hard to do what I ask."*[29]

Of course, she does not mean romantic or sexual love. This needs to be said to temper the panic button that has just been pushed by the health regulatory bodies. Dr. Meisinger refers to a reciprocal caring. She loves patients and patients love her back.

People will care for themselves if they feel cared for. What role can humanity and love play in helping people in need? As Dr. Meisinger says, caring for people is the work that health care does.

HUMANS, NOT HEROES

There is an unfortunate hero narrative in health care that is applied to doctors, nurses, and other health professionals. If you are labelled a hero, it is implied that you can no longer act as a human being. This means you must be perfect at all times. You can never do any wrong. You must save victims and you never have to look at them as people. You cannot have a bad day.

And you are untouchable. Nobody can criticize or provide constructive feedback to a hero, can they?

Anyone who works in a health care setting must be allowed to be human. The cult of perfection in health care is dangerous for professionals' mental health and the patient experience.

Heroes don't bother to connect with the people they are saving. They just swoop in and save them. Heroes don't create safe spaces for patients to speak up with safety concerns or feedback. They quickly shut that down. Defensiveness and guarding of the status quo by heroes are not going to create the change in health care that we desperately need.

I want a clinician who will show emotion when she discloses a difficult diagnosis. Who lets me peek into her heart. Who tells me a bit about herself. I'm not asking to be her Facebook friend. But if I know she has a toddler at home, this humanizes her and gives us a connection, something to chit-chat about before we get down to business.

Allowing me to see you as a human being builds trust because connection is the foundation for building a relationship.

Nobody is perfect. Dr. Jillian Horton's seminal book, *We Are All Perfectly Fine*, is the story of her experience at a mindfulness retreat for physicians. It is a stark reminder that the pressure to be perfect in medicine can break people.

Dr. Horton describes the culture of medicine:

> *"We are also compliant and conscientious and rigidly perfectionist, characteristics that put us at risk for choking on our own misery..."*[30]

Staff and clinician well-being has bubbled to the surface with COVID. It should have always been important, but now human resources departments are panicked about retention, as staff leave the health care profession.

The antidote to this is a reimagined world of health care, where people are at the core, not systems or executives.

"I began to feel the suffering of my patients more acutely...but also their strength and joy," says Dr. Horton, describing what attending the meditation retreat gifted to her.

The opposite of burn-out is not to depersonalize patients. It is to turn back towards them with an open heart.

While waiting for a system transformation that may never come, health professionals must turn inwards to care for themselves. This goes way beyond the self-care mantra of yoga and bubble-baths. I discovered this truth as a patient when I attended a cancer retreat a year after my breast cancer treatment.

I couldn't do anything to go back and fix my poor patient experience in the cancer hospital. I was carrying around all that rage and it was damn heavy. I tried hard to advocate for change for patients, but I was minimized and dismissed by administration. Pressure to advocate as a patient is a responsibility as heavy as a block of concrete.

My epiphany at the cancer retreat was that it was not in my control to cure cancer or improve experiences. It was in my control to carve a spot for peace in my heart. That meant putting blame, guilt, rage, and sadness aside, even for a moment. The peace comes from first recognizing how much we are carrying and then laying down of all these heavy burdens to take a rest.

Retreats for cancer patients and retreats for physicians have that in common: a search for inner peace.

Pretending to be perfect does patients no favours. Perfection blocks listening. Perfection blocks feedback. Perfection blocks patient safety. Perfection blocks health professionals from allowing themselves some grace.

Perfect breeds all sorts of unsavoury things: defensiveness, expertness, ivory-towers, patient-dismissing, gaslighting, mental health troubles, challenges working in a team environment, and undue pressure on individual human beings to get everything right. Perfectionism harms health professionals, those who work with them, and those they are supposed to serve.

I want my doctor to be able to say, "I don't know" or "I was wrong." With the explosion of medical knowledge over this past century, I know that health professionals can't possibly know everything. The notion of the country doctor who has the answer to all ailments has gone by the wayside.

It is a relief when my physician says – 'I just have to look this up. I don't know, but I will find out and get back to you. I will talk to a colleague first. I changed my mind. Let's consider a number of choices together. I'm sorry, I made a mistake.'

Uttering these phrases is freeing for everybody. It also helps health professionals forgive themselves when things inevitably go wrong. Even if you consider yourself perfect, you are not. Nobody is. Mistakes will happen whether you are a perfectionist or not.

Be humble, vulnerable, and show patients that you are human.

DO YOU VALUE ALL PATIENTS?

Do you value all patients?

When I say patients, I do not mean only patients who are people like you. It is safe to say that all health care professionals are college-educated, most are English-speaking, and very few – if any – are poor. Most staff in health care relate easily to patients who are college-educated, English-speaking, and not poor.

I have spoken to medical students about having a son with a disability. One of the first questions I ask them is: 'Do you know any disabled people?' Very few of them put up their hands. There is the rare student who has a brother or sister who is disabled (and perhaps influenced their decision to go into medicine) and a few who have volunteered with Special Olympics. The majority of students look at me blankly when asked.

Let's dig even deeper into this question. How many high schools have truly inclusive education programs? Where I live, children with disabilities (or 'funding' as they so eloquently call these students) are included in elementary school settings, but when they hit high school, segregated classrooms abound. Sometimes, the segregated class is even in a separate building.

My son Aaron went to 'regular' classes, but that was only because of persistent lobbying from his parents and an open-minded principal. Even then I am not positive that he was fully included in these classrooms – often times, he sat at the back with his Educational Assistant (EA).

Once Aaron and I spoke to a Leadership class in a high school, which was full of students – possibly future medical students – who were high-achievers. We prepared a talk to the class about Down syndrome. When Aaron got up to speak, most of the class looked very uncomfortable. Some of the students were looking at him like he had three heads. I asked if any of them had classes with Aaron and a couple of them put up their hands. It was clear that even though Aaron was in class with them, they did not know him. They were certainly not friends with him.

I wonder how many high-achieving, elite students are shielded – by the education system, by their families, through their own ableism or fear of people who are different than them – from disabled people. How many of those students go on to choose a career in health care?

True inclusion would support these future health professionals. If they got to know a student like Aaron, maybe they would think of him as a person instead of a diagnosis. Maybe they would see his strengths. Maybe they would even reach out to be his friend. This rarely happens right now in our school settings. Students bring their values to their post-secondary studies. If they aren't given the chance to examine their own biases, they will bring them directly into their health care practice.

It is guaranteed that people who become health care professionals will work with people who are different than them. They will encounter many disabled people, but they may not have any disabled people in their lives. How many medical students live in high-income neighbourhoods? Many families who have disabled children cannot afford to live in these types of neighbourhoods as they are often forced into poverty. This is for a variety of reasons including the lack of caregiver-friendly workplaces, long waitlists for accessible childcare options (that cause one parent, usually the mother, to leave the workforce), and the high cost of private therapies and equipment.

How many medical students go to private schools? There is little economic diversity with those who go to medical school.[31] Many private schools choose to not accommodate disabled students.

Even if they go to public schools, how many medical students actually get to know a disabled student in their school?

God knows we tried. We asked if Aaron could join an after-school club at the high school, but we were told no because the clubs were student-led and there would be no supervision for him. He was named the Most Valuable Player for his Grade 7 basketball team, so when he hit high school, he tried out for the basketball team. The team was clearly so competitive that he, of short stature and slower reflexes (although he can shoot hoops if he is given the chance), would not make the team as a player. We asked if he could be a manager. Again, we were told 'no' because the team was 'student-led.'

I'm drawing on our own family examples to make a point. If high school students see the education system devaluing students with disabilities, how do the students value people like Aaron? How does this feed into their own biases? What sort of exclusionary behaviours do they bring into college and subsequent health practices when they work with patients?

Getting to know disabled students would be a start. It would provide a peek into their future practice, where they might disclose a prenatal diagnosis. Or have someone with an intellectual disability on their clinical roster.

I'll ask again: Do you value all patients? This question should be posed to senior administrators too.

The public health COVID policies created by senior officials have been ableist and discriminatory. Vaccine distribution has been inequitable, both at the local level and globally.[32, 33]

Disabled people are at the back of the line for the COVID vaccine, despite the fact that they have been proven to be high risk to contract and die from COVID.[34]

How have the public health officials valued the people they have been serving? In British Columbia, the restaurants, hair salons, gyms, and ski resorts remained open throughout most of the pandemic. In fact, in early 2021, ski resort workers were vaccinated a month ahead of people with disabilities.

In some jurisdictions, schools were re-opened in September 2020 but were not safe for medically compromised students or teachers, so they were excluded and remained isolated in their homes.

It is hard for me to wrap my head around the fact that physician administrators have had a hand in making these discriminatory policies. Physicians who signed on to do no harm to all patients, not just patients who are elite and look like and sound like them.

Yes, politicians have influenced public health policy in many countries. My country's medical system is publicly funded, so that means that the government operates our health care system. Politicians lead the government so that means that politicians run health care. It is not a surprise that health care is political.

What is a surprise is that health officials have not stood up, demonstrated integrity, and refused to roll out discriminatory policies.

My son Aaron had the opportunity to ask a question to the Minister of Health at a vaccine Town Hall during the pandemic in March 2021. He asked:

"Do you care about disabled people or not?"

The Minister did not properly answer Aaron's question. We are still waiting for a satisfactory response.

JOY AT WORK

J oy at work is important and often forgotten in serious health care environments. I was a participant in a *Society for Injecting Humour in the Hospital Workplace* at a rehabilitation hospital many years ago. We held fashion shows and dance parties in the auditorium. Everybody was invited to the performances – patients and staff.

Humour is often lacking in health care. *Sickboy* Podcast is an exception – they promise and deliver a listening experience that is "hilarious, ridiculously insightful and absolutely determined to break down the stigma associated with illness and disease!"[35]

It is refreshing to hear the hosts' irreverent conversations about reverent topics. Their interviews about health care are honest, even if they are about painful subjects.

Joy *at* work is important but so is joy *in* work. I once had a position in a hospital where the staff morale was excellent. Staff described working there as being like part of a family. There were pictures of clinicians on the wall when one walked into the facility. People stood and chatted in the halls, and there were friendships nurtured outside work hours. Staff yoga was offered at lunch and there were craft sessions in the library during employees' break-times. There was a constant stream of employee social events – teas, skits, and barbecues.

I was hired to advise about patient-centred care. Many staff were offended by the very idea of me – of a person brought in to improve the patient experience. They felt strongly that they were already patient-centred. The staff were satisfied with their work family and wanted to keep it that way.

Despite the good morale, it was obvious who came first at the hospital: the staff. The culture was strongly staff-centred, which was not necessarily great for patients.

Patients shared feedback that they felt dismissed and not listened to. Patient complaints were often ignored, their voice mail messages left unanswered for weeks. Information given to patients was chock full of deficit-heavy medical jargon. Diagnoses were shared with patients in a dark meeting room with no windows, instead of the bright sunny staff boardroom downstairs.

"We know what's best for the patients," staff would tell me.

I spent months storytelling in an effort to encourage compassion. First, I told my own story about how it feels to be a caregiver in the health system. Then I engaged speakers who told their own patient stories. Along with the librarian, I started up a book club, where both staff and patients were invited to talk about books together like Ian Brown's *The Boy in the Moon*[36] and Anne Fadiman's *The Spirit Catches You and You Fall Down*.[37]

With a growing group of dedicated partners, we worked at recalibrating the focus of the hospital to include patients. I lobbied unsuccessfully to invite patients to the yoga class. I managed to replace the staff pictures on the wall with colourful art to better reflect the people who were being served and to change the first impression when people walked into the hospital.

I wasn't trying to take away staff morale; I was attempting to include patients in the staff's happiness. There's a difference between experiencing joy *at* work and feeling joy *in* work.

I enthusiastically agree that staff well-being affects patient well-being. If a nurse gets yelled at in the staff room, it must be very challenging for them to walk into a patient room and offer good care. Patient safety is at risk in hostile work environments. As a patient, you can immediately tell if staff are unhappy, through their demeanour, lack of smiles, or poor eye contact. This is absolutely not okay and makes for a miserable environment for everybody.

Some may say that patient-centred care has tipped too far to the patient's needs. Let us not forget that patients are the health care's very reason for being. Patients are the one thing everybody who works in health care has in common.

Relationship-centred care is a more neutral term. If we care about relationships between people, then we care about both staff and patients' well-being because one affects the other.

When patients are excluded from the culture of well-being in a health care workplace, additional suffering can happen. Patients can feel like uninvited guests in hospital work environments, as if they are a bother and an afterthought. I still feel like that when I go to the cancer hospital, apologizing as I check in at reception. The receptionist always looks up reluctantly, clearly annoyed at my presence.

I continue to champion staff well-being and shout about the importance of it from the highest mountain. This is both selfish – as a patient, I know that happy staff means better treatment for me – and because I do care about the health professionals in my life. Start with staff well-being, but factor in patient well-being too.

It is crucial to not forget about the patients in a quest for a healthy workplace. Staff and patients are tightly intertwined. As the tired pandemic saying goes: we are all in this together.

For health care staff, well-being is not just about experiencing joy *at work*; it is about honouring your greater purpose. Your greater purpose is the reason you chose health care to begin with, which is your *joy in work*.

Centre your practice on your purpose, and you will evolve from merely being happy at work to feeling deeply rewarded for doing what is perhaps the most important work of all: caring for people who are sick and suffering, who present to you when they are at their most vulnerable, often in the darkest times in their lives.

REFLECTIONS ON REFLECTIVE PRACTICE

L ike the intertwining of staff and patient well-being, staff and patient engagement need to happen at the same time. You cannot have one without the other.

Just like patients, staff must have safe places to tell their own stories. If they don't, they can hang onto their experiences in an unhealthy way. This in turn can interfere with demonstrating empathy and providing compassionate care. Telling your story can set you free.

In workplaces, sharing stories can occur informally between friendly colleagues, if one is lucky to have them. Organizations can contribute to a consistent environment of staff sharing through reflective practice programs, but simply instituting a program is not enough. Space for reflective practice must be given every single day, for all staff, not just for clinicians. Staff must feel safe enough to talk to their managers and each other about difficult situations, without fear of being judged or punished.

Reflective practice is sharing a story about something that happened, figuring out what you learned from it, and planning to do things differently next time. Sadly, reflective practice is rarely a priority in frantic workplaces. Being still and simply listening to each other is becoming a lost art, even between colleagues. All health

care workplaces expose staff to traumatic experiences, and therefore leaders have the responsibility to actively care for their staff.

Reflective practice can be adapted to any kind of work environment. Facilitating reflective practice sessions with those in caring
professions is one of my favourite things to do.

Culture will have changed when these types of conversations
occur naturally, every day, instead of waiting for a professional
development workshop to create a space for them.

 In group reflective practice sessions, start with an easy
icebreaker, ask roundtable questions like: What did
you have for breakfast or what's the story behind your
name? Once connection is established within a group,
work up to sharing the stories behind why people chose their
profession. This type of sharing really gets to the heart of why
people do what they do. Colleagues find out full origin stories that
go beyond where their workmates went to university and pieces
of hearts are slowly revealed.

Health professionals can naturally have challenges when working with stressed or angry patients. Facilitators must be careful
not to offer solutions and instead listen carefully and reframe
questions when needed. Sometimes I'll tell a bit of my own story
as a mom of a disabled child, or as a cancer patient, to provide a
different perspective. Often someone else in the group has a good
idea to share with their colleagues, so when that happens, I simply
listen and stay silent.

Many times, people know the answer to their challenges in their
own hearts. Sometimes people just need space to unlock it. Other
folks just observe and listen and that's perfectly okay too. There

must be sensitivity to this sort of conversation, and it should never be forced.

There are also formal reflective practice programs.

The Gibb's Cycle of Reflective Practice is a classic exercise taught in schools. It includes describing an experience, delving into feelings about it, evaluating it, analyzing it, drawing a conclusion and creating an action plan about how to do things differently next time.[38]

Other types of reflective practice are group-based programs, like Schwartz Rounds, which brings staff together to talk about the human dimension of health care, including feelings after difficult situations.[39]

Cleveland Clinic offers details about a Code Lavender model, where patients, family, or staff can call a Code Lavender when a stressful event happens in the hospital. Within 30 minutes, a Code Lavender team of spiritual care and healing services will arrive. It is described as, "creating space for conversation and crying," and while Code Lavender doesn't profess to prevent burnout, it is meant to "add to the healing environment of the hospital."[40]

Some may fear that reflective practices can devolve into venting sessions. There is nothing wrong with making space for venting. Health care organizations tend to shy away from negative feedback from anybody – patients and staff included. The key is to have a facilitator to help conversation move beyond the negativity into a reflection of what feelings it brought up and to make a plan in case it happens again.

In order to effectively engage in reflective practice, clinicians must get comfortable with sharing stories about their own experiences in health care workplaces. Only after that will they be open to disclosing their feelings about events. This is the hard part, for sharing feelings can make anybody feel vulnerable.

No matter what approach is used, the crucial thing is that people are given a safe space to share their stories and feelings, without judgement. Health care environments that dedicate time and space for staff to process hard things are healthy workplaces.

WE ALL HAVE STORIES

A t a talk with a group of Pediatric Intensive Care Unit (PICU) nurses I asked, "How do you take care of yourself when a child you are caring for dies?" They looked puzzled until one nurse slowly put up her hand and said, "Well, if we have a friend who is working that shift, we might talk to them about it. Otherwise, we are given a new patient assignment and told to get back to work."

This answer almost made me cry. There was no formal way on this unit – an intensive care unit, where children do die – for the nurses to pause in order to process their own grief about a child's death. It made me realize that there are three stories here: the child's story, the family's story, and the nurse's story. And all of these stories matter.

I have been very focused on patient and family storytelling over the years. It took a 16-hour trip across the ocean to Australia for it to dawn on me that *everybody* in health care has a story that needs to be honoured. I had been tightly holding on to the notion that it is *only* patient and family stories that need to be heard.

Patients and family stories matter, yes absolutely. And because of the massive power imbalance in health care, these stories are often ignored, minimized, interrupted, or dismissed. There is a considerable amount of catch-up that needs to be done so that patient and family stories are valued both at point of care and when decisions are being made in organizations. I will continue to beat on this drum.

But my unwavering opinion about stories shifted when I headed Down Under.

I had the opportunity to go to a series of events called the Gathering of Kindness to launch my book.[41]

The Gathering of Kindness aims to "build, nurture and instil a culture of kindness throughout the healthcare system," and is focused on staff well-being, not patients. Before I left, I had to think long and hard about the connection between patient stories *and* health professional stories.

Patients care about their clinicians. For patients to form relationships with health professionals in our lives, professionals must let us get to know them as people. This means allowing patients to see you beyond professional titles by sharing bits of your own story with those you care for. Patients need to know you before they can trust you.

If health professionals can understand their own stories in health care, this can help them heal from challenging experiences at work. Reflective practice hinges on sharing stories.

On top of reflective practice exercises, another tool is narrative medicine. A better name would be narrative health care, to not exclude those who are not physicians.

Narrative medicine is described as, "A Model for Empathy, Reflection, Profession, and Trust," by Dr. Rita Charon. It includes providing opportunities for clinicians to reflect on their work through their own writing and to read stories about the experience of illness to deepen their understanding.[42]

I saw Dr. Charon speak a few years ago. She was adamant that paying attention to stories helped clinicians to be totally present with patients.

Isn't caring for patients an act of humanity, and not a function of science? If health care really is about relationships, then the stories of everybody involved in the relationship must be considered carefully.

As Dr. Charon said, "Pay attention to where the suffering happens, for that is where the healing begins." This is true, no matter one's title or role.[43]

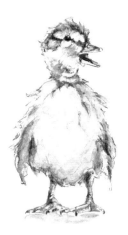

PART 3

HEALTH CARE REIMAGINED

L et us imagine the health care world we want to see. This reimagining is within our control. This section outlines ideas for staff and clinicians to spark positive change within their own realm of control. These ideas are for people who want to invest in a better health care world, one that is rooted in love and compassion.

A version of the Serenity Prayer, adapted from the 12 Step Program applies here:

> *"...grant me the serenity to accept the*
> *things I cannot change,*
> *Courage to change the things I can,*
> *and Wisdom to know the difference."* [44]

Individuals working or being cared for in the health system cannot change many things. Ordinary folks in my home country of Canada cannot adjust the funding formula for hospitals, which is based on a sickness model, not a prevention model. They cannot alter how many physicians are funded, which is through the fee-for-service model. They cannot change what types of health care are funded by the government – right now it is medical care, not mental health, not pharmaceuticals, not dental or eye or foot care.

There are many who have dug into these issues, like health journalist André Picard. His book *Matters of Life and Death: Public Health Issues in Canada*, tackles issues like 'policy gridlock' and unpacks the challenges of Canada's Medicare system, asking if we get value for our money.

"Our medicare is a relic, frozen in time," Picard concludes.[45]

Picard outlines gigantic system-centred problems. These problems are not unique to Canada. There is not one solution big enough to fix these messes. Health care administrators and their highly paid consultants love to use the terms transformation, quality assurance, change management, quality improvement, total quality improvement, lean, pilot projects, and innovation. Some change has happened because of these initiatives. But they are only incremental improvements.

The reasons for the problems are more deeply rooted. Trotting out an initiative or a pilot project to fix a broken system is akin to putting a Band-Aid on someone in the ICU.

Instead, let's pause to imagine the world we want to see. There are actions still in an individual's control, even under a broken system. If everybody committed to doing one simple act every day, like helping a patient who is lost in the hall or fetching a cup of coffee for a student, these acts would build and build until they became the norm, not the exception.

Just take one extra step. If you don't fancy yourself a rabble-rouser, support someone who is. This could be as simple as sitting beside a colleague who is sticking their neck out in a staff meeting for support or sending a thank-you email afterwards.

The problem is the elephant in the room, one that nobody except a few champions talk about: The health care system is not built on a foundation of love. The corporate health lens demands that health care is instead rooted in power, money, and efficiency.

Health care executives say they want change but what they really want is the status quo. Or such small, incremental changes that it doesn't touch them in their corporate offices, it doesn't reduce their salaries or risk their comfortable pensions.

The way to a new future is not to tinker with a system that is broken. Health care is not working for patients, families, staff, or physicians. Who is it working for? Those in the C-suites. Those who currently hold the power and who do not want to give it up.

There are three actions in this Health Care Reimagined section:

1. Climb down from your ivory tower to **be closer to the people.**

2. **Nurture safe spaces** for constructive feedback in order to learn and take action.

3. Lean on the **magic of the humanities** to put the humanity back into health care.

I offer these as Big Ideas, leaning on storytelling from my own experience in hospital workplaces, to show you practical ways you can embrace these ideas and turn them into real actions. I include references so that if an idea is appealing to you, and you want to learn more, you know where to look.

Dr. Victor Montori has written a book about the Patient Revolution called *Why We Revolt*. In it, he shares the actions of Dr.

Mark Linzer, a physician leader of general medicine at Hennepin County Medical Center.

> *"He slowed the pace. He stabilized the teams. He lengthened patient visits. He cleaned up and decluttered the walls. He simplified policies and helped managers see the time clinicians were spending caring for patients. He reduced waste caused by confusion, distrust and noise...he reminded clinicians of their calling. He showed them how each patient was a suffering comrade."* [46]

At a practical level, I've been involved in many projects within hospital settings. They included patient councils, book clubs, rewriting complaint processes, and creating more healing physical spaces.

I did not do this alone. I had the autonomy granted from my employers to be the dancing guy, and others eventually joined in. I hung onto the champions who signalled they would one day like to dance with me. They visited me in my office or accepted my offers to have coffee or a walking meeting outside the hospital. They wanted more care in health care too, but weren't ready to start dancing yet.

The key word here is that 'eventually' some folks joined in. Many times, I would be presenting my family story at a meeting and the staff audience would be looking at me like I had three heads. I'd go home and ask my husband: 'What am I even doing here?' and then get up the next day and continue on.

This work is mostly about being the dog with the bone, persistent in not willing to let go of the notion that health care can be a more caring place for everybody.

ENGAGEMENT IS OUTREACH

How to See People

A children's hospital once hired me to engage the families.
Engage the families whose children had been sick.
Engage the families whose children had died.
I was not foreign in their land.
I did not sit behind my desk.
I did not send emails.
I did not tell them to come to hospital meetings.
Instead, I went to them.
I climbed down the ivory tower,
Left the bricks and mortar,
And crossed the threshold past the parking lot,
To coffee shops and kitchen tables
For that's where the people are.

The families are already engaged
But just not with you in your business suits.
They are busy sharing lemon loaves and lattes,
chicken sandwiches and hot pots of tea.
And stories too, if only you will listen.
A guest in their honourable lives, I learned:
You will only see people where they are.
Not where you are.

For you cannot see a mother at a boardroom table.
You can only see her lying on a quilt on her living room floor
Beside her little baby, gently giving him breakfast
Through a tube that has been inserted into his soft belly.

WE ARE ALL EXPERTS
IN SOMETHING

For 16 years I've been involved – in both paid and unpaid roles – in what is now called Patient Engagement. There are stories of patient engagement that go well and there is patient engagement that goes badly.

Like patient-centred care, meaningful engagement means partnering directly with patients, not doing things to them or for them. The first step is to respect patients' and families' time, experience, feedback, and wisdom.

I was invited to a meeting to talk about a hospital's new website. A family, a dad, had also been invited. It was fortunate that he worked in web design and knew about accessible websites.

It was a gift to have him there. He had prepared and shared a list of problems with the website – how the chosen colours made it difficult to read for people with vision challenges, how the navigation made it impossible to find anything, how the front page was full of corporate rhetoric, and didn't include the most important information, like where to park, a map of the hospital. Basically, the website had not been built to consider their most important audience – patients and families.

I sat in awe of his insight and suggestions. We all eagerly turned to the organizer of the meeting – this is great advice! How can we apply these learnings?

"Well, my hands are tied," said the chair. The communications representative had not shown up to the meeting so the chair could make no decisions.

"There's nothing I can do without her here!" the chair continued, throwing up her hands. Our faces all fell.

"Um, could we have another meeting with her to discuss? Could you bring these great recommendations forward?" I asked. There was a shuffling of paper and no answer. We uncomfortably looked down at our hands.

The meeting was adjourned, and we never had another conversation about the website. Tokenistic for the dad who had taken time off work to come to this meeting in the middle of the day? Absolutely. Tokenistic for the rest of the staff who actually wanted to make the website better for patients and families? Yup, it was a waste of time for them too.

I felt like leaning over to the organizer and shouting: "You are embarrassing us! Your hands are not tied! You have free will and influence! If you wanted to move this forward, you would! You have wasted this dad's time and he has so carefully prepared for this meeting!"

I chickened out and didn't say any of those things, knowing that making a superior look bad was the worst possible thing you could do in that organization. In this way, I was complicit too. I gathered up my things and walked out, profusely thanking the dad in the hall for their time. A few days later I emailed the organizer: Any follow up from this meeting? I never heard back. The website remains the same, six years later.

Patient and family representatives can make real change in the hospital world, if only the hospital leadership will allow it.

Years ago, when Wi-Fi was relatively new, a manager was advocating to the Information Technology (IT) department to allow families to access free Wi-Fi. This was in the early 2000's, when phones and devices became a common way for families to communicate with the world while their child was in the hospital. There was Wi-Fi available for clinicians, but none for the public.

The manager had been requesting Wi-Fi for years. She'd called countless meetings with the IT staff, which ended up being futile.

The IT staff kept saying there were privacy issues and risks that the public would access inappropriate websites using the hospital's network.

Finally, a dad on the family council got wind of the struggle. He happened to be an IT consultant and understood how to talk to IT folks in IT language.

The manager and the dad requested another meeting. They listened to all of the IT department's barriers, the reasons why they kept saying, 'No, it can't be done.' The IT dad structured the conversation to provide the facts so that there was no way for the IT department to keep saying no.

The IT staff had been confusing the hospital staff with all their mumbo-jumbo. The dad understood this and acted as a translator for the clinicians. He addressed each barrier as it came up.

Finally, the request for Wi-Fi was brought to the senior director of privacy for a signature. This director worked in a corporate environment, far away from patients and families. But he was a dad too.

The IT dad met with him, and politely asked, "How would it feel to have one of your kids in the hospital, but to be unable to communicate with any of your family while you were there? You wouldn't be able to provide updates as to how your child was doing or bring your laptop to do some work so you wouldn't have to take as much time off."

The senior director paused and thought for a moment. Then he signed off on the request.

Patients and families bring their own expertise, whether it is at the point of care or at the organizational level. The first step to building an environment of relationship-based care is recognizing and respecting this expertise. They know themselves, their bodies, and their illnesses well, plus they come with personal and professional experience beyond being a patient.

The dad in the first story was dismissed and there were no positive changes made to the website. In the second story, that dad was listened to, leading to action that benefitted patients and families.

Patients and families bring their own expertise, and they are a help, not a hindrance.

START HERE FOR
MEANINGFUL ENGAGEMENT

Let's move past being well-intentioned to actually doing patient and family engagement right. If you don't evolve beyond intentions, you're not only doing nothing, you may even be causing harm to people with your misguided efforts.

It is common to have staff teach patients about patient engagement. This is backwards. Yes, patients and families can always learn more about the medical system, but, in most cases, it is the staff who need training on how to engage with patients – and patients should be the ones to facilitate it.

There are many people who have worked on credible, non-corporate resources for those who want to do patient engagement right, starting with the Patients Included movement, founded by Lucien Engelen.[47]

"That there should be so much talk about what patients need and want without them being present prompted me to take action." says Engelen.

Patients Included offers charters for organizations to make sure they don't exclude or exploit patients. Charters are written by patients themselves, and detail best practice to include patients in conferences, patient resource materials, journals, and ethical discussions.

Patient engagement's sister, patient-centred care, includes organizations like Planetree, The Beryl Institute, and the Institute for Patient and Family Centered Care. All three offer resources and professional development about patient-centred care and patient engagement.[48, 49, 50]

The Gathering of Kindness was started in Australia, and partners with patients to improve staff – and ultimately patient –

well-being.[51]

"We are on a mission to get patient experience evidence taken as seriously as medical evidence." The Patient Experience Library in the UK offers fantastic articles and references for practical patient engagement.[52]

In the Patient Experience Library's Inadmissible Evidence report, they outline the harm inflicted on patients when they are not listened to, along with ideas for solutions: formally collecting patient experience information, not dismissing patient feedback as 'complaints,' formalizing patient experience roles in hospitals, learning from adverse events, and respecting patient stories as much as medical evidence.[53]

One note of caution – do not lean exclusively on organizations and their resources. No organization, including patient organizations, speak for all patients, although many say they do.

The best resources are outside your door – the real patients and families who use your services. But do not treat them merely as resources. They are people who come with stories, trauma, and wisdom. If you reach out to the people in a meaningful way, you will be surprised what magic might happen.

KITCHEN TABLE REVOLUTION

Patient engagement positions are outreach positions.

This work is not about sitting at a desk behind a computer, sending out emails to patients, telling them to show up to focus groups or committee meetings in the hospital boardroom. A hospital centred approach like this, adopted by so many organizations, misses the point of engagement.

Patients and families are not the same as staff sitting in their cubicles, refreshing their email and waiting to be summoned to meetings. They have lives outside the hospital. They are at work, or picking kids up from school, or, ironically, at the hospital for their own medical appointments. Maybe they aren't feeling well or they don't have the resources to take time off work to attend a daytime meeting, or they don't have a vehicle to get to the hospital, or going to the hospital causes anxiety and stress because they've been traumatized there.

I have been invited to dozens of meetings – maybe over a hundred – as a patient or family member. Only a handful of them were held outside of the hospital walls. One was on the hospital campus at a university building. A few others at private golf club settings – presumably so the senior executives would be most comfortable?

None of these meetings were held where the people are – at community halls, libraries, or coffee shops. Or in the kitchens and living rooms of the patients themselves.

Few patients or families want to return to the hospital. Even putting aside the trauma that is inflicted in that environment, parking is notoriously awful and expensive. Hospitals are often located in the middle of pricey neighbourhoods near where physicians live, not patients and families.

For instance, the new children's hospital in Vancouver is smack in the middle of one of the most expensive neighbourhoods in the city. I know of no families who live nearby, but plenty of specialist physicians who walk to work. If the hospital had been truly family-centered, it would have been built out in the far suburbs where the families can afford to live.

There is power in the kitchen table revolution. The secret sauce to successful patient and family engagement is to engage people where they are at – both mentally and physically.

When I worked at children's hospitals, I went out into the community because that's where the people are. I dragged clinicians out of the hospital to meet at nearby coffee shops because that's what regular people do. I'd encourage walking meetings, where we talked while strolling around the hospital grounds instead of sitting at a meeting room table.

The environment in the hospital is stifling in so many ways. There are constant overhead pages announcing codes. People are rushing from place to place, overly busy, their heads down looking at cell phones. This is not a place for creative thinking. Until culture changes, it is an environment fraught with committee meetings, tasks, and routines. Hospitals think they are corporate entities, with their business suits and minute-taking, but this is a lie. Health care facilities are merely the bricks and mortar vessels for delivering care to vulnerable human beings.

Dr. Don Berwick, former President and Chief Executive Officer of the Institute for Healthcare Improvement has a book, *Promising Care*, that reprints many of his speeches over the years. There is a lot of gold in this book.

> *"Change will happen...when we realize that our*
> *white coats and our dark suits are disguises...our next*
> *big step is to not just serve people but to join them."* [54]

Leaving the hospital to meet a family at a local café is a way to shed the white coat and business suit. The only business health care should be in – particularly in publicly funded systems – is the business of caring and serving other people. Exit the hospital and meet people where they live, where they work. The hospital is an artificially constructed environment ripe with power hierarchies.

Location, location, location. If we recognize that there are power imbalances in hospital environments – between patients and staff, between staff themselves – then we know that even walking into a hospital setting adversely shifts the power imbalance against patients.

Patients have to find childcare, book off work, locate parking, pay for parking, and then find the meeting room. When we are in the meeting room, we are often outnumbered. One family told me of showing up to a meeting as the only family representative, and sitting in the boardroom alone, waiting for the staff participants. The hospital staff all showed up late to the meeting, and had obviously stopped at the coffee shop together, as they were all toting Starbucks take-away cups. The meeting had not even started and she felt excluded.

Lest you think this is minor, these 'little things' are actually 'big things' and symbolic of the beginning of an engagement relationship.

Once I was invited to speak at rounds for a physician specialty group with two hospital staff members. We were told to show up at a specific time in the middle of their meeting, which we dutifully did. The meeting room door was closed. We knocked on it tentatively. Someone opened the door a crack, annoyed that we had interrupted them. The little room was packed full of physicians.

'We aren't ready for you yet,' the person hissed, and we slunk away to sit in the waiting room. When we were called back in, there was nowhere to sit. Nobody made room for us – it felt like we were a massive intrusion to the meeting. I can still remember the feeling of awkwardness standing uncomfortably in that crowded room. Reluctantly, some folks began to shift chairs to make space for us, their guests. After we presented, we were summarily dismissed and we slipped out, grateful to be done.

Adjusting behaviour to be a good host does not take a lot of effort.

How easy would it be to do these things for meetings?

1. Ask someone to be the assigned 'host' for guests or newcomers.

2. Meet up with guests at an easy-to-find hospital entrance and walk to the meeting room together.

3. Consider getting together before the meeting time to chat about what to expect and to get to know each other so there's a familiar face at the meeting.

4. Offer to stop for a coffee if it is the culture of the group to bring their own coffee to the meeting.

5. Find a chair for the guest and sit beside them. Casually introduce them as people come into the room and include them in the informal 'chit chat' of the group.

6. If there's technology involved, make sure someone is there to get slides set up, microphones turned on, etc.

I can't tell you how many meetings I've arrived at as the invited guest speaker where nobody is responsible for the technology. I'm standing at the front of the room with my USB in hand and everybody in the room shrugs – 'I don't know how to turn on the projector,' while I'm frantically plugging things in and trying to log on and pushing buttons while everybody is watching me. I immediately start sweating. These simple problems add stress to the poor speakers who are probably already anxious about public speaking.

These are important things that can be done to create a welcoming and comfortable atmosphere for your guests before the meeting even begins. Consider being creative about where you are asking people to meet. Even better, ask people where they want to meet. You might be surprised by their answer.

HOW NOT TO ENGAGE

One evening, I attended a Models of Care presentation at an acute care hospital. My son had been a patient on the nursing unit that was changing their models of care. (To this day, I'm not even sure what a model of care is).

The meeting was held in the windowless basement of the hospital. I seem to spend a lot of time in windowless meeting rooms.

I arrived at the appointed time, and the room began filling with tired-looking mothers. After the roundtable introductions, I realized that the organizers had gone up to the nursing unit and recruited families who had children actively on the unit – children who were acutely and sometimes gravely ill – and asked them to come to their meeting. I can remember the exhausted faces of the mothers under the buzzing din of the florescent lights.

The organizer gave a presentation about Models of Care. Unfortunately, this was the same presentation she gave to clinicians, and I did not understand one word of it. There were acronyms and lingo – and despite my English and Health Administration education, it was way over my head, even as a rested mother with a well child.

When it came time to give feedback on the model, the mothers from the unit shared their stories about their children. How they became sick, the trauma about being admitted into the hospital, the lack of sleep and services. One mom said, weeping, 'nobody is taking care of me.' The issue of caring for the mental health of families when their children are hospitalized came up over and over again. The organizers nodded grimly, making notes on their clipboards.

These families were clearly brought in, taking time away from their sick children up on the nursing unit, to put bodies in chairs in that dim meeting room. Were they at a point in their health care journey to reflect back on some strategic initiative like Models of Care? No, no, no. Hauling them downstairs in their sleep deprived, stressed state seemed morally wrong. Many of them cried in that basement boardroom, with nobody to support them or give them a hug. It was an awful train wreck of an engagement attempt gone terribly wrong.

Afterwards, I asked the organizers what kind of feedback about their models of care they received. Was it what they were hoping for?

"No," they said bitterly. "All the families could talk about was their own experience," they said. "They didn't give us any useful feedback."

I am still angered at this lack of awareness of the harm they caused these parents in their quest to get their participation numbers up. They had not done the work to build relationships with families who had past experience at the hospital.

THE HIJACKING OF
PATIENT ENGAGEMENT

Two decades ago, patient engagement was in the patients'
hands. Councils were formed from grassroots groups of patients,
families, and caregivers. Over the years, as the influence and power of these groups grew, the organizations stepped in to take over.

The health bureaucrats have hijacked patient engagement.
Patient engagement portfolios are headed by anybody other than
patients themselves. Positions in patient engagement are post-
ed as full-time jobs, often with a graduate degree as a minimum
requirement. This professionalization of patient engagement work
automatically disqualifies most patients and families.

The problem with this approach is that a full-time position does
not work for many people who have chronic conditions or who
are caregivers of kids with disabilities or medical needs. Requiring
a graduate degree is another red flag that the position isn't accessible to patients or caregivers, who hardly have the time, nor the
money, to pursue advanced education.

Hospitals are not looking to hire someone who has a different
perspective from their own staff. The irony is that patients and
families are not outsiders – they are insiders. As peers of patients
and families, they have excellent skills to engage others. Having a
layperson perspective on health care is essential if you want your
ducks in a row.

Patients do not need someone in a corporate suit to represent
them on their behalf. What was once an organic revolution,
concocted in living rooms by regular folks over pots of tea, has
been stolen from patients and families. It is just another health
care administration job now, handed to a Vice President as a soft,
non-clinical portfolio often when they have one foot out the door

heading to retirement.

A hospital executive once asked me: do patient engagement positions always have to be filled by people with lived experience? There are many good people working in pediatrics who do not have children, or folks who work in adult health care who have never been a patient.

Yet not making patient engagement positions accessible for patients means they don't even get a shot at the job. At the very minimum, positions should be created equitably so people with lived experience can be considered for them.

An accessible position offers flexible hours, allows work-from-home, minimizes unnecessary meetings, gives autonomy to meet outside hospitals, provides a focus on the delivery of work instead of the hours clocked, and does not demand a graduate degree for qualification.

Consider: does your patient engagement approach validate the status quo or does it venture into innovative territory? If you want change, you must change the ways you do things. The same old way is going to get the same old results.

MY OWN WORK STORY

The first time I did direct family engagement for a pediatric hospital was as a volunteer. I was invited to sit with another mom on a panel, interviewing candidates for the position of Manager of Family Centred Care. This was before the concept of hiring a patient to do this job had even been born.

This was an all-day affair. Once again, I got dressed in my business suit to look legitimate, and we sat in yet another windowless room hosting interviewee after interviewee. Upon introduction of the panel, four of the interviewees expressed shock that there were two moms sitting there looking up at them. One interviewee, Heather Mattson McCrady, exclaimed upon meeting us, 'Of course there are family reps here!' and so it was not a surprise that she got the job.

The magic with Heather is this: she is passionate about this work, and she is an exceptional, non-judgmental listener. Her education includes an undergraduate degree in recreation administration and a master's degree in theological studies. More importantly, she brought the values needed to excel at this job. Skills and knowledge can be acquired; values cannot.

She recognized that this work was more like community development – that is, creating a movement for change – as opposed to developing a program. Heather acknowledged everyone's part in creating change and that each person brought forth their own passion, skills and wisdom into the mix. She says that magic moments are made of this combination:

> *"Patients and families were the catalysts that created a resonance of passions, along with management and staff, to ultimately influence hearts, change behaviours and actions, and benefit the care and health of children and teens in health care."*

Recently, Heather was asked what her secret was to family engagement. 'Well, to start, I had Sue Robins by my side,' she said thoughtfully. Now, this is less about me, and more about having a model of a staff member working together with a family leader. We were peers. She worked from inside the system, listening and looking for opportunities where the family and patient voice could influence change. I ventured outside the system to engage with families, as much of my work was to extend goodwill out to them from the hospital.

There were many initial steps in the early journey. We first had a Planning Circle with family reps and senior leaders, physicians, and staff. It was held off-site to get everybody's head out of the hospital, away from the distractions of overhead announcements and inboxes. We brought in an external facilitator to run the meeting. In our prep meetings with her I was stubborn and resolute: we must get a commitment to begin a council, I said, or the whole thing is a failure.

The day unfolded like a strategic session. Participants shared what family-centred care meant to them, what the hospital was doing well and what they could be doing better. Towards the end of the day, we still didn't have a commitment to begin a council. I cornered the facilitator in the women's bathroom. She was a sweet and skilled woman. 'We must get the commitment that we will start a council,' I said, feeling desperate as it was getting late in the day, and the leaders were dancing around the issue.

Back at the boardroom table, the facilitator asked directly: 'Do you commit to starting a family council?' There was a pause and some hesitation. 'Yes, I commit to starting a family council,' the chair answered. BOOM. Those were the words we needed to hear, and we were off and running.

There were many steps to establish a family voice in the organization. The secret sauce contained many ingredients. As Heather focused on staff engagement, she was visible at management meetings, to connect with other leaders.

I was a broker of goodwill between the hospital and families. Thankfully, from my work with community groups in the disability world, I knew a lot of families. Family leaders were identified by staff, and I adopted my mantra: 'See you, know you, like you, trust you,' and made it my mission to get out and connect with families everywhere and anywhere I could.

Heather used to joke that 'Sue is going for coffee again.' I was thankful not to have an office at the hospital. Instead, I had dozens of meetings with families in coffee shops. I broke a lot of bread over lunches with family leaders. If families had young kids or childcare issues, I went over to people's homes, bearing take-away coffees when I knocked on their doors. I sat on the floor and played with kids, joined them around the kitchen table and ate muffins. Basically was a regular mom – as opposed to a health care professional – because that's what I really am.

Change happens in health care when the grassroots rise and the senior leadership is open and ready to join them in this revolution. Patients are knocking on boardroom doors, demanding change. It is a leader's job to consider if they are going to unlock the door and let them in.

Five years later, I accepted a new position at a pediatric rehabilitation health centre in a new city and a new province. I uprooted our shrinking family – our eldest kids had been launched into independence – to be the hospital's Family Advisor, which was a brand-new position. Contrary to the sound of the title, I did not advise families. I almost exclusively advised staff – that is, the staff who wanted to be advised by me.

Early on, I met with a respected therapist. I was struggling to explain my work, which is an unconventional mix of storytelling, creating opportunities for families to contribute to decisions, and extending out to people in the community.

'I educate staff about family-centred care,' I offered, and was met with a stern look and rebuke. 'We don't need to be educated about family-centred care,' she said, angrily. 'We are already family-centred.' I heard this refrain over and over. We don't need you because we are already family-centred.

From this, I learned about the importance of using the right language with staff. Even the fact that I had been hired to advise about 'family-centred care' was offensive to some staff. If they were already family-centred, why did they need a Family Advisor? Good question. I lobbied to change my title to 'Family Engagement Advisor,' which helped temper this defensive response.

I slowly began to meet families. I drove all over the west coast to meet them close to home. Once I drove up the beautiful highway along the ocean to meet a family leader in an independent coffee shop. Afterwards, we strolled down Main Street and she took me into a fabulous chocolate maker, and I stocked up on little exquisite chocolates to bring back to work. Another time I drove east for an hour on the busy highway in the pouring rain to take a mom for lunch at the mall. I met a mom in her small apartment in the city and another mom in her basement suite in the suburbs. I picked up sushi and brought it to a dad and his family to share a meal together before a big stressful meeting. A mom whose son was on the inpatient unit was having a hard time, and I managed to steal her away and we met up for French food at a little bistro.

Most of these conversations were about real life, not hospital life. We got to know each other as people, not as roles or titles.

I drew heavily upon the peer support training that I had taken when I coordinated a program for families who had babies with

Down syndrome.

I learned numerous things about visiting families in their homes. I took off my shoes at the door. I accepted snacks or beverages that were offered to me. I recognized the value of chit chat to break the ice. I was excited about meeting their children, and truly delighted in holding the babies.

Mostly, I sat and listened. This I learned from Heather – the value of sitting and holding space with a family to listen. Heather's studies in theology and spirituality taught her that, and she in turn taught that to me. I hugged families and I cried with them too. I brought out my own story only if it was relevant to share, and then I put it back away and listened to the family story. I never interrupted. I answered a lot of questions with a gentle: 'I don't know.' It was okay not to know. I wasn't there to fix. I had one job and that was to listen to understand.

It was essential to focus on the most important question of all, which is: 'How might I feel if it was me?' You will never know how it will exactly feel if it was you, but you can draw upon your well of empathy to demonstrate compassion. The best family advisors understand that sympathy is not the same as empathy. Sympathy is pity, sympathy is patronizing, sympathy is condescending. People can sniff out sympathy from a mile away. I'd rather someone be rude to me than feel sorry for me because I have a child with a disability. Empathy is more equitable. It is being open enough to feel what the other person feels, without judgment. Empathy shows that you care.

Patient engagement work is not about you, my friends. You must check your ego at the door. It is about first creating opportunities for patients and families to share their stories and wisdom. And then supporting staff and clinicians to learn from this wisdom and then affect positive change in their practice and behaviour.

Storytelling is a key component of this, for people communicate with each other through stories, not through data or research. Health professionals love data and research. But laypeople don't communicate in numbers. They communicate with words.

What, pray tell, does a paid Patient or Family Advisor do?

Most of my work was supporting storytelling. I coached speakers and prepared audiences to be open to listening to stories. These stories can take many different forms: presentations to staff at Grand Rounds, opening meetings with stories, speaking at staff meetings, talking at staff orientation about what's important to patients and families, and teaching medical or other health faculty students.

The important part is to integrate these stories into existing speaking opportunities as well as having special 'patient-centred care or partnering with patients' events. If you only have patient-centred care talks, only the organization's champions will show up, and you will be preaching to the converted. If stories are included within existing professional development time or staff meetings, then all staff become exposed to stories.

The next question to ask is: Whose stories are being told?

THE D WORD

For a decade, I attended a national children's conference. On the program every year was a panel about diversity.

In the early years, the panel would be stacked with so-called experts of mostly white clinicians. Later, a single person would be included who had lived experience with racism in health care, but they were outnumbered on the panel by people who were anointed experts in diversity and inclusion.

The topic of diversity was repeated year after year. Clearly nothing ever changed. It was like watching the movie Groundhog Day on repeat.

Whose stories do we value? Hospitals complain that they don't have diverse patient engagement from people who are 'marginalized' but don't realize that they are the ones who have marginalized them. People in these communities are not inherently hard to reach. You just haven't tried hard enough to reach them.

This is true in research too. A book called *Understanding and Using Health Experiences* says this, "Remember the 'seldom heard' or 'socially excluded' groups. Don't use the term 'hard to reach' because it suggests the problem with engagement lies with the groups, not the researchers."[55]

As a white middle-class woman, I will not be talking about diversity in patient engagement in health care. People in my demographic have been standing behind the podium for a long time. I will hand the microphone over to Patient Leader and mom of three, Amy Ma. She graciously shared her wisdom for this chapter.[56]

"There is a lack of self-awareness that you inherited a system that you benefitted from. That's called privilege," Amy says. It is important for people associated with health organizations to recognize that they are white-centred.

"Don't ask the oppressed group to educate you on a problem they didn't contribute to," she continues. "It is a waste of our time and energy to console you."

If you are uncomfortable reading this, good. Feeling uncomfortable means you are growing. Keep reading.

"There needs to be a recognition that the health system does real harm to people. There is racism here in Canada, even if we are more polite and subtle about it," Amy continues.

Amy's wish is that people would educate themselves about their nation's history, which includes their own health profession. Florence Nightingale had a role in British colonial violence and Dr. William Osler, who has been described as a "Saint in a White man's dominion," regularly offered up racist comments about people living in Latin America as well as Black and Indigenous people.[57, 58]

Health care needs to first reckon with the skeletons in their own closets, says Amy.

"We need to look at all of our histories: the good, the bad, and the ugly, beyond the hallowed halls of academic white men," she advises.

It is a lonely space for Amy to be in, as a racialized woman and a Patient Leader who champions diversity and inclusion work.

> *"I walked into my first meeting at a children's hospital in 2013 and looked around to see if there were any visible minorities or disabled people in the room. Seeing Indigenous and Southeast Asian people there made me feel like I was welcome to join."*

Her advice for councils and committees is to observe who is missing and identify the barriers to their participation. This means reimagining patient engagement and to shift it towards community engagement, in order to meet people where they are. "There's been a lot of talk lately about increasing diversity and inclusion around the table, but maybe we have to rethink the whole idea [of gathering people around one table] and meet them on their terms, in their territory," says Amy when she was interviewed by the Canadian Medical Association Journal about engagement.[59]

Amy gives examples of how community engagement can happen. Cosmetologist Tessie Bonner has a powerful story about her work raising awareness about breast cancer with her Black customers in her salon.[60]

Amy describes another initiative to reach taxi drivers about the risk of diabetes. Knowing they couldn't come to an information talk in the evenings because of their long work hours, organizers went to the taxi drivers instead, sharing information as the drivers waited for customers at the airports between flight arrivals.[61]

Diversity includes people with disabilities too. Amy shares that some Patient and Family Advisory Councils, like the University of New Mexico Hospitals, have a budget for a sign language inter- preter to include deaf and hard of hearing people on some of their committees. The Ottawa Hospital has a Deaf Patient and Family Advisory Committee (PFAC) that is focused on QI (Quality Im- provement) initiatives. The co-chair of the Deaf PFAC also sits on the Corporate PFAC.

My own son Aaron has been asked to speak to the media or at health conferences, but he asks for modifications so he can be suc- cessful. Instead of appearing live at an event, he submits a pre-re- corded video so he can practice what he wants to say.

Amy believes that change often comes from the fringes and from autonomous organizations, not from inside the health care system.

"This push towards the professionalism of patient engagement means that organizations are requiring master's degrees to apply for a job. This qualification is a tool of oppression – it is exclusionary and causes gatekeeping," she tells me.

She explains how health care's paternalistic model means people in health care have a vested interest in keeping the status quo going, instead of creating meaningful change.

Amy encourages diversity as far as social class too, and that all patients deserve to have their experience validated.

"What about the single mom who has a child with the medical appointment, who works shifts, has a hard time taking time off work, and struggles to afford gas and parking to get to the hospital?" Amy asks. We cannot forget about these patients.

"What side of history do you want to be on? Those who oppress or those who liberate?" Amy asks.

Despite the slow progress, Amy is still hopeful for the future. "My children know more Indigenous history than I did," she says. "Even a land acknowledgement is a start. We have to begin this work by having conversations." It begins with going out to the community to engage with the people.

Amy has generously shared several resources, which are in the Notes at the end of this book.

It is the responsibility of those who are in privileged positions to do their own research about diversity and inclusion. It starts with me and it starts with you.

TWO STEPS BACKWARDS

Patient and family engagement took a hit during COVID, but it was slowly sliding backwards even before 2020. Councils were being disbanded. Patient and family staff members were resigning or being forced out, and then their positions were filled by clinicians.

Replacing patients and families with clinicians swings the pendulum back to 15 years ago. Professionals are now speaking for patients instead of creating environments where patients can speak for themselves.

Why has this regression happened? I can only speculate, as the research on patient engagement is sorely lacking. I believe that as paid patient and family advisors become more vocal, administrators become threatened by their influence. The advisors' honest feedback about health care makes professionals increasingly uncomfortable, and these new positions take away the patient power.

Patients should be accepted unconditionally, including if they are outspoken and angry. The pressure to be a compliant patient is strong in health care – whether it is at the point of care or organizationally. Wisdom should not only come from well-behaved patients.

There is a real fragility that underlies the patient engagement movement. If patients and families behave themselves, then all is fine. The minute there is a change in leadership, or something gets hard – like a pandemic, ethical issue, or conflict – then boom, it is over.

This movement is so precarious that it can only survive when things are going well. I define going well as when patients and families mirror their behaviour as closely as possible to the behaviour of clinicians and administrators. We must dress like them, talk like them, show up when they tell us to, and agree with them. Of course, this erases any hope for diversity and leaves the pool of engaged patients as university-educated, articulate, and economically well-off individuals, just like the clinicians and administrators themselves.

Patient engagement quickly becomes doomed the moment there's a sniff of any difference or contention.

The past five years, there has been a trend in many health organizations to replace paid families or patients with health care clinicians in patient engagement roles. This is obvious from the job descriptions, which are full-time, in-person positions that require graduate degrees. These types of rigid jobs are not accessible to most patients or caregivers.

What happened to the notion of offering flexible positions that encourage patient and caregiver applicants? The patient engagement movement has become too successful. We have amassed too much power in the eyes of administrators. This, ironically, means that engagement has become no longer tokenistic and is finally meaningful. But to have power you must take power – and administrators and clinicians aren't willing to give their power up.

Paid family members and volunteers are not 'professionals' (nor should they be, especially if people are truly looking for diversity), but health care is built on the structure of professionalism. Having laypeople without graduate degrees make decisions in ways that are not tokenistic is just too much for many bureaucrats.

The way patients and families are treated at the organizational level mirrors the way they are treated at the point of care. If there is bad morale and low patient satisfaction at the bedside, then efforts in patient engagement at the organizational level will suffer too (and vice versa).

Many people in senior leader positions do not understand the role of patients in organizations. They might understand the bedside engagement, but the patients in organizations concept is new and poorly understood.

Health care culture is also exceedingly slow to change to new ways of doing things. Patient engagement shakes the status quo. In the health care system, the status quo does not wish to be shaken.

Patients in paid positions on councils or committees do not have a common job description, standard training, or defined core competencies. In other words, they are not regulated in any way. The health care environment is one that demands structure and regulation. There should be standards and support, but not in a way that puts people in a rigid box. This work – which is outreach work – needs to remain nimble and creative.

Patient engagement still butts up against some professions and threatens them. I'm thinking of those clinicians who think it is their job to advocate for patients, not the job of the patients and families themselves.

This regression has been compounded by the COVID pandemic, when organizations dropped patient engagement like a hot potato. The lack of meaningful engagement was obvious in 2020 when a strict 'visitor' policy was enacted in hospital and supportive living settings.

Back in 2009, Kingston General Hospital was one of the first adult hospitals to enact a flexible visitor policy, recognizing that "family, friends and other support members contribute to positive health outcomes and a positive patient experience." [62]

Other hospitals followed suit, some even abolishing the concept of visiting hours altogether.

Visiting restrictions came screaming back during COVID, leaving 17-year-olds alone to fend for themselves in adult Emergency Departments. A disabled person, Ariis Knight, who had cerebral palsy, was left alone to die in the hospital in April 2020 with no means to communicate. The wife of a man with dementia was escorted out of a hospital for daring to hold her husband's hand. Many people died alone in ICUs without their loved ones at their side.[63, 64]

In the early days of the pandemic, there was little consideration of the idea that visitors are essential care partners and no effort into finding ways for them to be at their loved one's bedside in a COVID-safe way. There were also risks to not having family presence, which led to increased anxiety and patient harm. The notion of essential caregiver slowly began to take hold.

Healthcare Excellence Canada defines an essential caregiver as, "An essential care partner is a person who provides physical, psychological, and emotional support, as deemed important by the patient or resident."[65]

Restrictive visitor policies are a symptom of the fact that patient engagement has fallen by the wayside. The pandemic has exposed many truths, including the fact that patient engagement was fragile to begin with. There's a long way back to rebuilding trust and relationships between people and organizations.

THE ART OF REALLY LISTENING

Once you reach out, then what? For outreach to be successful, it starts with listening.

> *"The best sort of people are those who create space for stories. They can sit with an uncomfortable story without minimizing it, interrupting, looking for the bright side, correcting the storyteller or running away."* [66]

Before you even get to listening, you have to create a safe space for people to tell their story. Safe spaces have to do with trust. Why should a patient you've just met trust you and feel comfortable telling the truth? Is it just because you are wearing a hospital lanyard?

In the treatment room or the boardroom, patients are often asked to tell the story of themselves, but the story too often has to fit exactly into health care's narrow template of what a patient narrative should be.

This is hard stuff; in some ways, harder than memorizing the Krebs Cycle. [67] That's why calling interpersonal skills 'soft skills' is so ridiculous. Working with people is much harder than knowing facts. Perhaps it is time to stop equating soft with being easy.

Once a safe space has been created, the right questions need to be asked to get the story rolling. Don't ask the wrong questions. One pet peeve of mine is being asked if I had prenatal testing for my now-adult son with Down syndrome. I'd much rather health professionals focused on the health issue happening today, rather than something that did or didn't happen 18 years ago. [68]

Be value-neutral and careful with your words. Be truly present in the moment. Don't interrupt the telling of the story. Let the patient know you are listening by sitting at the level of the patient (don't have a large barrier like a desk or a computer between you), make eye contact, minimize distractions, ensure privacy – and smile and nod. See? That's a lot.

This applies to one-on-one conversations in a clinic room or when listening to a patient speaker at an event. People asking questions at health conferences are notorious for only asking a question to show the audience how smart they are. Once I was at a health conference when an audience member asked a parent why they thought their child should get funding to receive a very expensive life-saving medicine. At another speaking event, a student asked a speaker how the death of her son affected her marriage. I cringe when I think of these questions.

There are a number of aspects to listening. Listen to understand. Don't listen with the intention of only thinking about what your response will be. Similar to reading comprehension – are you listening to what the speaker is really saying, or are you just hearing the words? This isn't a boxing match. You don't always have to respond with a counterpunch, a fix, or an answer.

Making space for listening takes longer and might be more uncomfortable than one thinks. A psychologist once taught me to ask a question and then sit in silence for ten full seconds waiting for an answer. Ten seconds seems like an eternity, so she suggested tapping out ten seconds on the roof of my mouth with my tongue while I waited.

Importantly, how a question is asked matters. She suggested instead of saying: 'Do you have any questions?' changing it to 'What questions do you have?'

> *"When we avoid an important topic, we miss an opportunity to strengthen that alliance."*
> *– Dr. Jon Hunter.*[69]

Health professionals can be reluctant to ask anything about the patient beyond a checkbox of medical issues because of a worry about opening a floodgate of emotions. Many clinicians don't fancy themselves as mental health professionals, so they can be reluctant to hear anything except for the facts about symptoms and lab results. They are concerned that if the box of secrets gets cracked, even a little bit, they will be sitting there for two hours in a makeshift therapy session. Let's look at the research about listening and empathy from the book called *Compassionomics*.

> *"In a busy outpatient clinic, researchers measured how long it takes for physicians to hear and respond to patients when an opportunity for compassion arises. On average: 31.5 seconds."*
> *- Stephen Trzeciak, MD, MPH* [70]

31.5 seconds. Listening, believing patients and acknowledging what they are saying can take very little time. Giving space to tell the story patients need to tell and then listening closely may in fact save time later on. Maybe if a patient does need two hours with a mental health professional, you could help them find the support they need? Perhaps other parts of the patient story, beyond the medical, are important to their overall health – so mental health is actually in everybody's lane too?

If nothing else, listening will start to build a connection based on trust, for all good relationships in health care begin with a foundation of trust.

Listening to understand is the way to honour a patient and their story, whether it is at the bedside or in a boardroom. Here's the thing: for me as a patient, feeling seen, heard, and validated, even for a few seconds, is priceless. That is why the story listening is just as important as the storytelling.

Go forth and listen.

THE NUTS AND BOLTS OF IT

P eople who work in patient engagement often ask, "How do I find patients?" Patient engagement done well is not merely about recruiting warm bodies or an exercise in matching a patient to an engagement opportunity. Patient engagement should not function like Human Resources departments or temp agencies. Going out to the people, knowing patients as human beings, and allowing yourself to be known, beyond your title, helps form true relationships.

Health organizations do not necessarily need formal patient engagement programs to partner well with patients. It is enough to have one champion who believes in the power of the patient voice, who wants to have a patient on an interview panel, who hires patients as editors for patient materials or asks them to speak at staff orientation, although there's no denying that a budget to do this work helps. This is not 'side-of-the-desk' work.

There are two practical steps in engaging patients: First is forming that relationship with them. This takes time and requires trust. The second step is how patients are treated once they become involved with an organization. Relationships are more than just the wooing. You don't lure someone in for a first date and then treat them like crap afterwards. That's tokenism. This betrayal is worse than not even involving patients to begin with.

There are many ways to meaningfully include patients in an

organization. It is not only *what* you do to engage, but *how* you conduct yourself during the engagement. Are patients used and then discarded? The only way to know if this has happened is to create safe spaces to ask patients directly about their experiences being engaged. The most valuable type of feedback often comes from patients who withdraw from opportunities, so don't merely ghost people after the opportunity is over.

THE SECRET SAUCE – ENGAGEMENT 101

Patient-centred care, patient and family-centred care, patient engagement –whatever you want to call it, I'm talking about health care staff, physicians, and systems relinquishing power. This power shift is needed not just to give patients an equitable voice, but for patients to finally step in to lead their own health care. This chapter is for you if you believe in authentic patient engagement at an organizational level.

I reflect on my learnings from my years working at a children's hospital, where families and staff worked together to build a family council from scratch.

First, have integrity. There must be an alignment of professed values and actual behaviour. If your mission statement says Patients First, then the behaviour of your organization, through its policies and processes, must be Patients First every single time. This philosophy should also be evident in the actions of all staff too.

This means doing serious self-reflection on how you treat all patients and how you handle feedback, even when it casts a bad light on the organization. You cannot say you are patient-centred and then roll your eyes at 'difficult patients' or 'hysterical mothers' or dismiss patient feedback and the stories that you do not want to hear.

The only people who can say if an organization is patient-centred are the patients themselves. Management cannot arbitrarily decide this and slap buzzwords all over their website as some sort of PR exercise.

Integrity means that if you say you want to hear the patient's voice, you make space for the uncomfortable stories and honour those who tell them to you. Listen hard and don't turn away.

Seek out your most unhappy patient. Make the time to create a safe space, listen to understand and take action on what they have to say. Their feedback is a gift to you. This is Quality Improvement in action.

If you want to collaborate with patients in a meaningful way, you must be willing to give up your power. Patients are vulnerable in health care settings. At the bedside, you have to concede some of your control and do everything you can to minimize their trauma and suffering.

If you want patients around your boardroom tables, then you must make room for them at those tables and treat them like equals. That means not pulling stunts like scheduling meetings last minute, demanding people volunteer their time, or not preparing or debriefing with patients.

Giving up some of your power, you also must admit that you can't and don't know everything. Being an 'expert' is the ultimate patient-centred care killer.

Creating opportunities at point of care for patients to safely speak up and share their wisdom helps them heal. It also helps them connect with one another to build their own community. Oppressing and dismissing stories and feedback harms patients. Ask yourself: do you want to heal or do you want to harm?

Magic can happen when staff, patients and families are in alignment. If you really want to put patients first, the first step is to sit down and be humble.

THE CONSULTANT WITH
THE EXPENSIVE SHOES

When my son was three, I was asked to attend a strategy session for the hospital where he received rehabilitation services.

I was excited about being invited and I had an endless amount of input to share about our experience at the facility. I understood strategy development from my professional life at the Department of Health and as a board member on our local Down syndrome society, so I felt I had something meaningful to contribute.

I arranged and paid for an afternoon of childcare for my youngest son and for my other two kids to be picked up from school. There was no written material sent in advance, all I had was the start time and the meeting room number.

I drove to the hospital, paid for parking, and spent time finding the meeting room – which was tucked away in the basement of the hospital. When I arrived, the room was filled with families of pediatric patients and some former patients from the adult side. Some of the adults had caregivers with them. There was nobody from the hospital there – just a well-dressed woman at the front of the room, who introduced herself as a consultant. I knew she was well-paid by looking at her expensive shoes.

The next two hours were spent answering general questions about where we, as families and patients, thought the hospital's direction should be going. I was watching the consultant and noticed she took no notes at all over the two hours, which was awfully strange to me.

Afterwards, I asked her if I could receive a copy of the draft strategy for review, or at least a final copy for my files. I wanted to see how our comments would be incorporated into the document.

"Oh, yes, I'll email you a copy" said the woman with the expensive shoes. I didn't see her write down that request either. You probably can guess what happened next.

We were thanked for our time, ushered out, and I never saw a copy of the strategy – draft or otherwise.

Now, this was only a few hours of my life, but it was a red flag for my future involvement at that facility. I persevered in participation – presented to a senior management group about family-centred care, talked to clinic staff about family experience, and I also sat on their parent council as a volunteer for four years. But that hospital never really 'got' what meaningful participation meant, or how to engage families.

Meeting times were often set arbitrarily and with short notice, without consultation of family schedules, presentation times changed last minute, and nobody ever met with me beforehand to prepare. I was just told to show up. When I got there, I often was not introduced to those around the table, and that felt very intimidating to me, as a Mom. I finally gave up and faded away because I felt my voice was not being heard.

The antidote to tokenism is meaningful engagement. Let us redo this engagement in a meaningful way.

The consultant had a list of stakeholders she needed to confer with – including families and patients. Inviting the stakeholders to the strategy session was only one step. How were participants chosen to attend? Was there diversity of experience in the invitees? Were patients even involved with planning the strategy session?

Then there are logistics. People do not always want to return to the hospital for meetings. Why not consider locations that are closer to where the people are instead of expecting them to come to you?

She should have documented the session and meaningfully listened to the participants. Patients and families also needed to know that their feedback had been incorporated in some way, and if it wasn't used, the reasons why.

To close the feedback loop, the draft strategy should have been circulated to the stakeholders for review, or at least, the final product should have been shared with the families and patients.

The consultant did none of the required actions to make the experience meaningful for the stakeholders. This resulted in a 'Check Box Phenomenon', where the consultant only ticked a box off her list after meeting with patients and families and had no intention of incorporating any of their feedback into the hospital strategy.

Taking a few steps back, tokenism can also occur even before a strategy session takes place. If families and patients are brought into the information collection process too late, and the content of the strategy has been decided by other stakeholders, then their feedback is rendered meaningless.

The secret to meaningful engagement is two-fold: first, build meaningful relationships with those you wish to engage with, then strive to flatten the hierarchies that are inherent in the health system.

WORK IS WORK IS WORK

I got a silly idea in my head after my cancer treatment was done. I thought – well, I've taken a break and now need to get back at it. I applied for a patient position on a committee with a research group at our local health authority.

For this volunteer position, I had to fill in a long application form and go in for an in-person interview. My first interview was re-scheduled at the last minute by the organizers. I showed up on the second interview date and was told: "One of the interviewers is running late. Can you come back in an hour?" I wandered up and down in a nearby mall for an hour and then returned, nervous I wouldn't be finished in time to pick my son up from school.

A physician and an executive director conducted the interview. We were crammed into a small windowless room. (By now, you can see that the windowless room is a theme in my patient engagement career). I tried to cheerily chit-chat, but they were having none of it. I don't know how many alarm bells I needed before I actually got up and left.

The interview was intense and formal. It was as if I had applied for a management position instead of a patient partner one. Towards the end I brought up the concept of compensation. Everybody else on the group was getting paid by their employer to sit on the committee, everyone except for the patient. I had done my research and knew that similar committees offered compensation to their patient partners.

A bizarre back and forth followed:

Me: I know that other committees offer the patient partner compensation. Will you be doing the same?

Executive Director: We considered compensation, but this is a volunteer position.

Me: But if you don't offer compensation, you will not get diversity in your patient partner. Not everybody can afford to work for free. You will only get representation from privileged people like me.

Executive Director: (Looks at me blankly). We decided if we pay patients, it will seem too much like work to them.

I blinked a few times, processing this answer.

It was clear that they did not want diversity. They wanted people like them – who were wealthy enough to work for free. I gave them a tight smile, thanked them for their time and made my exit. When I got an email a few days later, telling me I had been appointed to the committee, I turned them down.

This Patient Experience Journal article thoroughly explains the concept of patient compensation: "...marginalized populations are confronted with financial and social determinants that are often barriers to full inclusion."[71]

If the concept of patient compensation is difficult, consider this question: should staff be paid? If the answer is yes, then patients should be offered compensation too. Otherwise, this adds to the power imbalance between patients and professionals.

 The answer is to incorporate patient honorariums or fees when planning the budget. Talk with patients to see what rate is fair. Know that some people won't accept monetary compensation for their own reasons or require alternative compensation. Be flexible when offering pay, and have the conversation at the beginning of an engagement, not the end.

It is awkward to talk about money. The best relationships in life involve two people who take the time to talk about uncomfortable things and make decisions together. These relationships can exist in patient engagement too.

WAITING ROOM EXPERIENCE

When nothing in health care feels easy, making small adjustments to physical space is a good place to start.

I wrote about the importance of first impressions and waiting rooms in *Bird's Eye View*. The phrase 'waiting room' shows up 47 times in my book. Obviously, the waiting room is an important element in my patient experience. While waiting rooms are often overlooked, they are complex environments. A lot happens there, including a first impression. If a first impression is bad, you can never get it back.

> *"The majority of patients arrive in health care settings in some sort of distress. Why not first welcome them into the clinic or hospital? Why not install signs that say the word welcome in many different languages to create a positive first impression?"*[72]

First impressions matter. They set the tone for the rest of the interaction. The physical space of a waiting room seems like a fairly easy thing to change to make it more patient-friendly. There are many aspects to a waiting room: has it been built to welcome everybody through universal design? What is the aesthetic, including what's displayed on the walls? And how are people treated in the waiting room?

Once I toured a children's hospital's waiting room with a mom who had a daughter who used a wheelchair. We walked into a clinic that had chairs lined up against the walls." "Where is my daughter supposed to sit?" the mom rightly said. There was no room for a wheelchair or other mobility device like a walker. The child's wheelchair would be blocking the aisle. This was not a welcoming environment for this young patient and her family.

There are ways to fix these physical problems and they have to do with universal design. This means designing waiting rooms so that they work for everybody. Talking to patients and families about their ideas to improve waiting rooms would be a great first step. They have good solutions because they spend a lot of time waiting in waiting rooms.

These places should be healing environments. Replacing the tattered signs taped up on the wall with artwork would be a good start. Consider playing soft music to create a more peaceful setting. These are simple changes that can make a big difference.

A pre-admission clinic at a children's hospital has volunteers who sit on the floor and play with young patients and their brothers and sisters while they wait for their appointments. This is a thoughtful gesture, and both amuses the kids and allows the families a bit of a break from tending to their children.

Another clinic has a little fridge that contains snacks in the waiting room. Patients and their families are welcome to help themselves if they are hungry or thirsty.

When the concept of offering snacks was brought up to administration, they responded, "Well, people will abuse this and steal the food." The answer back from the staff was, "If people are hungry or thirsty when they come to our clinic, shouldn't we simply give them food?" The resourceful clinic manager went to the foundation to make a pitch for a snack budget – and voilà! – the clinic now offers sustenance to people who are hungry.

The waiting room process can be softened too. It is like purgatory to sit there and wait for an unknown period.

 Some clinics have instituted systems that release patients so they can go grab a coffee or go for a walk until the doctor is ready to see them. This can be done simply by handing out restaurant-style pagers that go off when it is time to be seen, or by using electronic tracking methods online, so you can see when your number comes. Even restaurants now text your cell phone when they are ready to seat you. Surely the health system could learn from the restaurant industry about improving the waiting experience. At the very least, could there be an indication from the receptionist about how long the wait might be?

As I said in my first book, I am often cranky, stressed and anxious when I enter a health care setting. I wonder if some of my bad mood could be mitigated by simply being welcomed into a peaceful environment. It strikes me that less cranky patients would help everybody – patient, families and staff too.[72]

Thinking carefully about first impressions would help get the health care relationship off to the right start. Even before people arrive at a physical space, there is a first impression that comes with booking the appointment.

Can patients book their own appointments online or by phone? I often felt I was at the mercy of a booking clerk during my cancer treatment.

If appointments are booked by phone, are booking clerks friendly? Do they offer options or are patients just told when to show up? Is there an easy way to follow up? Are options given for communications preference – by text, email, or phone?

Are patients told to show up early and then forced to wait for an indefinite period? This is one of my pet peeves. The considerations for scheduling should take into account that the patient's time is important too.

Are people told how long they should expect to wait? I was at a pediatric dentistry appointment with my son and a receptionist came over and apologized for the wait. She explained why there was a delay and gave us a sense of when my son would see the dentist. She asked if we needed anything and suggested we had time to go grab a coffee. I almost fell out of my chair. This courtesy has never been extended in the publicly funded health care world.

There's lots involved with the wait. Are patients given support when they are waiting for an appointment to be booked? Told details like bus routes, parking information, and directions? Are there extended hours at clinics for those in school or at work?

If this seems overwhelming, pick one single thing to work on.

Go and sit in the waiting room. Do you enjoy sitting there? What do you see and hear? Start with looking at the visual clutter. Often there are signs haphazardly taped up all over the walls. Are the signs friendly? Translated? Is there a way to merge some of those signs? Are the signs replacing communication with a real live person? (They shouldn't be).

Consider privacy. Can you overhear staff on the phone or talking to patients at check in? The receptionist at my oncologist's office is famous for making personal calls for all to hear. This shows a lack of consideration for the anxious cancer patients privy to her carefree social plans.

Look at your physical space. Is the receptionist desk up high, which immediately creates a power imbalance and is not accessible for people who use wheelchairs or those of short stature, including children? Are the chairs in the waiting room welcoming for people who need bigger spaces to sit or are they constrained by the arms of a chair? Is there somewhere to lie down if people are feeling rotten? Is the sitting area friendly for people who use wheelchairs or other mobility devices or are the chairs lined up in a grim row, with no spots for a wheelchair or even a stroller?

Think about what there is to do while waiting. The local diagnostic imaging place has a sign taped to the wall that says 'no cell phones allowed' but everybody ignores it. Magazines have disappeared because of infection control, but is that really a valid reason? The only thing I looked forward to when my daughter was at the orthodontist was reading the brand-new magazines left for parents in the waiting area.

The waiting room at the cancer hospital features a loud blaring television that was always tuned to CNN. My radiation treatment unfortunately coincided with Trump's election, so I was subject to a horrible montage of Trump's audio and visual for 20 days.

I soon figured out that the television was for the staff, not the patients. Staff would wander past to stand and watch the news as all the cancer patients sat hunched waiting for our appointments.

This is hardly a relaxing environment.

My favourite spaces are ones that don't have a television at all, or if they do, it is turned to a nature channel that features soft chirping birds, not Trump rallies.

Ask yourself: Is your waiting room a welcoming and healing place?

 If you'd like patients to be prepared for their appointment, offer a pen and blank notepad for them to write down their questions. Consider the barrage of health information in waiting rooms – pamphlets, health education TV shows – is that what patients want or is that what clinicians want? I don't know that answer. Ask the patients.

It matters what happens to patients after they arrive. Often, we have to fill out paper forms on clipboards with information that we've already shared.

Sometimes we are given a number and then a receptionist yells out our number. It does not feel good to be referred to as a number. I am not a customer in a deli.

How do patients move about in the environment? Are patients moved from space to space (which is disruptive) or do staff come to patients who are settled in a comfortable room?

This is a lot but it becomes manageable if you break it down step by step. Wondering what patients want from their waiting room experience? Just ask them. Waiting rooms are a good place to start.

CHECK YOUR WALLS

I walked past photographs that lined the walls of the cancer hospital every day I had treatment. They were not photographs from patients – rather they were the results of a staff photography contest. Could there really be anything more provider-centred than staff-submitted photographs on the hospital walls? Physical space does speak to the culture and priorities of an organization.

I worked in a children's hospital that had a similar decorating style. At reception, there were black and white photos of staff doing therapy to patients. This was the greeting when you walked into the building. At least it represented the work done at the hospital, but it was also terribly provider-centred in a different way. The pictures were about thirty years old, so I had my excuse for a refresh.

There were two champion staff members who backed me in my mission to replace the photos – one a clinician who herself had been a patient in her youth and who understood the notion of patient-centered care. We had heard anecdotes from families that the photos were not welcoming, so I embarked on a project to replace them.

Some stars aligned for this art project. The hospital foundation had a room full of original paintings that had been donated to the hospital. It just needed some coordination to choose paintings and to get them installed. But first I needed to get the old photos off the walls. That was my challenge.

This hospital employed many staff who were working there in the 1990's when the photos were taken and installed on the walls. The staff were fond of their pictures and were wary about my plan to refresh the artwork. I called it a 'refresh' as opposed to 'get rid of those old pictures' for obvious reasons. I had to think of a solution that was also staff friendly.

I began to investigate who was in the photos. I enlisted the more senior staff's help to identify the children and the people in the photos. By involving them at the beginning, this helped me gain support. As a coincidence, some of the staff were retiring. I suggested presenting the photographs as a gift at their retirement parties. I emphasized we had free, donated art to refresh the walls. There was some grumbling, but this seemed okay.

There were about 18 pictures in total. There were five photos with current staff in them. I went to each staff member individually and asked if they wanted the picture themselves, or if they wanted me to track down the child in the photo and ask their families if they wanted it, or if they wanted their photo placed up on the wall – in a place of honour – in another part of the hospital. I let them decide.

I know some staff were unhappy with the change. I received a furious email from a nurse who had worked at the hospital for over 35 years. He let me know I was disrespecting the staff. I asked to meet with him to chat but he never responded. I continued to be friendly with him in the hallways, but he shot daggers from his eyes and avoided me. This was a hard lesson in being disliked for being a champion for change.

I continued on. We had an art show with the new paintings for the families and staff to provide input and get used to the idea of replacing the pictures.

Upon reflection, I cannot believe the effort it took to get those damn pictures replaced. This is a window into health care culture. Change is often fought tooth and nail, even if it is positive change.

Switching the pictures that had hung on the wall for almost 30 years ended up being a big project. This whole thing took months. No wonder nobody else had tackled it over the years. I believe in polite persistence. I kept on going with a smile on my face. I had leadership behind me, my two champions and feedback from families, so I kept moving forward.

In the end, the old photos were replaced with child-friendly, stunning original artwork from donors to the hospital foundation. When you first walk in, there is a huge colourful polar bear by the front reception. As you sit on the bench, there is a painting of a mother holding a baby. Other paintings are abstract, some more cartoon-ish – we used diverse paintings to represent the diverse group of kids served there – from toddlers to teenagers. I personally disliked one huge painting we ended up getting – a massive canvas of Tigger, but I had that installed on an inside wall and found that it was often used for wayfinding purposes ('turn at the Tigger'), which ended up being a good thing.

The paintings say to families and children when they enter the building: This is your place. We are a guest in your lives. Welcome.

Distributing the old pictures took even longer. They sat in my office for months as I figured out who was in the picture and then asked what they wanted me to do with the photo. Many of them got shipped to their rightful owners – some children who were now grown up, others to families whose children were in the photo, but had sadly died, others to staff who had moved on. Once I got permission and an address, I took the photos home and my husband and I wrapped them up in bubble wrap and duct tape for their safe shipment. We had wrapping supplies scattered in our living room for many weeks.

Take a look at the walls in your building. What do they say to the people who come through the doors? If you have authority to change them, use it. If you don't, try to influence those who do.

This ordeal was a lesson in many things: perseverance, change management, and selling an idea. It mostly taught me that if you want something done, stop talking about it, gather your supporters and get it done.

WAYS TO BE – OR NOT TO BE – TOKENISTIC

Thinking of engaging patients in your health
organization? Here are ten proven right and wrong ways
to engage patients.

1. Focus Groups

    Wrong Way: Inviting patients to your one-off focus
    group. I despise the term focus group. These words imply
    that patients will be engaged once and only once, probably
    late in the process, and their suggestions will likely be
    discarded. Those highly paid consultants with expensive shoes
    often facilitate these sessions. I also call this the Check Box
    Phenomenon.

    Right Way: Invite patient representatives to regular meetings,
    not just one-shot focus groups. Strive to communicate updates
    with them regularly, and sincerely ask for feedback that you
    then consider and incorporate. Engagement is not just one-way
    communication – it needs constant dialogue and collaboration.

2. Everybody Is Not a Patient

    Wrong Way: Assume that people who work for support
    organizations represent all patients. I call this the
    professionalism of patients, and I've witnessed this at
    conferences, where I sat on a patient panel of five people and
    was the lone patient. Everybody else was a paid staff member
    of a consumer organization.

    Right Way: Consider the purity of the grassroots patient voice.
    Staff representing patients always have a bias towards their
    organization's agenda. Think about how you define patients.

3. Speaking on Behalf of Patients

    Wrong Way: Have your corporate executives, clinicians, and researchers speak on behalf of patients, or be the lone voice talking about patient engagement or the patient experience. Don't do this, ever. It is exceedingly insulting to all patients to speak on their behalf and not make space for them to speak for themselves. This totally smacks of tokenism.

Right Way: Set a standard that there are no patient experience or engagement presentations without patients being meaningfully involved. They should be on the organizing committee and engaged as paid speakers and co-presenters.

4. Over-Volunteering

Wrong Way: Ask patients to over-volunteer. Have only a handful of people that you continuously call upon and expect them to show up at your organization for meetings numerous times a week.

Right Way: Your network of patient partners should be high in numbers so you have great capacity and diversity. Create sustainability in your pool by equitably sharing opportunities so patient reps don't experience burnout or bitterness. Consider going to the patients on their own turf – in their own homes and communities – and do not always expect them to come to you.

5. Relying on One Voice

Wrong Way: Hire a paid patient representative to speak on behalf of all patients, in all forums. The n = 1 model of representation is not diverse. Having one person present to health audiences, be the patient voice on committees, speak on behalf of all patients, is just plain wrong.

Right Way: Having a paid patient staff member is awesome. Use that person's role to engage more people and build relationships, so that you can bring forward multiple voices in the organization. This builds sustainability and allows for diverse perspectives.

6. Patient Engagement Conferences

   Wrong Way: Host Patient Engagement Events with no patients. Or, fly in a celebrity patient speaker from another country to deliver the opening presentation and pat yourself on the back for being so darn patient-centred.

   Right Way: Nurture your local talent pool of patient speakers. Yes, this might take some work. Coaching and supporting speakers who have experience close to home will create a more relevant and engaging message for your audience.

7. Expect People to Work for Free

   Wrong Way: Invite patient speakers to your conference or educational event. But don't offer to pay for their time, expenses, or registration. Pay all other speakers a fee and reimburse them for their time and expenses.

   Right Way: Show patients that you value their time and wisdom as much as health professionals by not expecting them to pay out of pocket for anything and consider offering a reasonable fee to cover their time.

8. Constructive Feedback

   Wrong Way: Ask patients to sit on your Advisory Council, but when they have constructive feedback you don't like, ignore that feedback, don't address what they have to say, and silently pave the way for their bitter resignation.

   Right Way: Patient reps aren't cheerleaders. Expect to hear feedback that you don't like, and respect that feedback by listening to it, responding to it, and collaboratively making a plan for how to improve things in the future.

9. Common Courtesy

   Wrong Way: Invite patients to participate in your organization, but expect them to show up on short notice, with no prep beforehand and no debrief afterwards. Give them an obscure room number and expect them to find their own way. Don't pay for their parking. Don't introduce them when they arrive in the room.

Right Way: Patients have families and lives. Give them lots of notice for meetings, and options to choose from so they can arrange childcare and take time off work. Patients are sometimes not well themselves. Plan for that by having a backup strategy (perhaps two patient reps, not just one). Extend courtesies to them. Pay for their parking. Meet them in the lobby and take them to the meeting room. Facilitate roundtable introductions when they get there. Take them for coffee afterwards to debrief.

10. Supporting Storytellers

Wrong way: Patients are paraded in to tell their story without any direction or coaching. This reduces the speakers to mere entertainment, or a tool to get an emotive response from the audience.

Right Way: Recognize that patients are sharing personal and intimate stories about their health with strangers. Honour the patient story by providing a listening ear, information about the audience, direction about key messages, and tips about public speaking. Support patients to succeed.

One final note on eliminating tokenism. Waiting until your organization has all their ducks in a row before you engage patients is the wrong way. The right way is to acknowledge that you will never have all your ducks in a row. Human beings are messy and health care is not perfect. Patients know this reality better than anybody. The time to meaningfully engage patients in organizations is now.

LOW HANGING FRUIT

I tried many things to create healing spaces when I worked at a children's hospital. Some ideas took flight while others crashed and burned. The key is to keep trying, even if it feels like your ideas are small. If one idea fails, move onto the next one. Seemingly small ideas can build and build to create big differences to patients. There may be ideas you can bring forward that are within your locus of control that won't put you in conflict with the bureaucracy.

A talented Indigenous artist was once waiting in the clinic waiting room with his grandson. I chatted with him about creating custom art for the dank waiting room and excitedly took his business card. I lobbied the managers and directors, but nobody would champion funding that project. That was a shame, since many of the patients were Indigenous and the artwork would be a sign that the clinic was a friendly one.

I attempted to make the library space more family friendly, but I was unsuccessful convincing others of the importance of this space. After my request to open up the library to families, the staff ended up locking the doors and having restrictive hours instead. The space ended up being more family unfriendly.

My effort to make the library more accessible to families had the opposite effect. In this case, a suggestion made things worse rather than better. Upon reflection, I think my great idea was a threat to the person who worked in the library and I had not engaged her well. She saw the idea as a threat to her status quo and built a brick wall to stop me.

I advocated to have the lunchtime staff yoga sessions opened up to families. Staff weren't interested in sharing their yoga time with families so that never took off either. Yoga seemed to be a sacred space for staff, and one person told me it was when they could take a 'break' from families. This is a sad reflection on the barriers put up between staff, patients and families. Yoga, of all activities, could have been seen as a safe space to come together as human beings. But it was not meant to be.

There have been many glimmers of hope.

Staff had their own ideas to be more family-centred, but until I began in my position, they had nobody to share them with. An Occupational Therapist came to me and asked, "Can you do something about the family kitchen on the inpatient unit?" I wandered down for a look.

Families on the unit often lived with their children, sleeping in uncomfortable beds by their sides. There was only one shower for all of the families, and they had to walk down the hallway past a strew of offices to have a shower.

Families took solace in the family dining room, eating side by side with their children. The kids were served food from the hospital cafeteria, and their families brought in their own groceries and made use of the limited cooking utensils. When I first saw the kitchen, the stove burners were filthy, the rice cooker was broken, and all the plates and cutlery were mismatched.

'What is the kitchen missing?' I asked one of the families using the space. A mom who had a child on the unit helped me create a list to properly stock the kitchen.

I went to the hospital auxiliary meeting one evening to pitch the idea of renewing the kitchen supplies. Their mandate was patient comfort and they recognized the benefit of families sharing meals together. My request was approved, which led to a field trip to a department store to replace everything in the kitchen.

A mom volunteered her Saturday afternoon, and along with my husband and son, we cleaned out the whole kitchen and restocked it, shiny and new.

This project gave me great pleasure. As a mom, I knew the power of cooking and breaking bread together. The least the hospital could do was to make sure the quality of the dishes and appliances in the kitchen reflected how we felt about families: not that they were broken and worn down, but that they were worthy of the shiny and new.

We also tore down the dozens of signs that were haphazardly taped up on the walls that said, 'Don't do this! Don't do that!' and replaced them with two signs that had positive language for the families: 'Welcome to your family kitchen. Please treat it like your own.'

The librarian in the hospital had a cousin who owned a local coffee shop. He generously donated coffee, and staff took turns stopping at his shop to pick up bags of coffee to stock the kitchen.

Start where you are at and evolve from there. Don't wait for everything to be perfect to begin.

The staff also led a few projects on their own. The conference room where they met families to deliver diagnoses was dark and dreary. A physician brought paint chips from her own home renovation project and the group arranged to get the room painted a lighter, cheerier colour.

This simple project led to a bigger one. The staff improved their workflow process to walk with families to the front door after their appointment was done. The paint colour change led to something more significant – a family-friendly way to wrap up an appointment and provide more time for families to ask questions.

Low hanging fruit should just be a start. Once those are picked, you can reach higher up on the tree.

These seemingly small initiatives are not that small at all. They accumulate to contribute to a welcoming environment for patients and families. Projects that include physical space or patient comforts are low hanging fruit. These quick wins are tangible and can be seen by staff. If a small project is a success, this paves the way for bigger initiatives.

The *Putting Patients First* book has a wealth of information and practical tips to create patient-friendly health settings. It includes case studies in the chapter called "Healing Environments: Creating a Nurturing and Healthy Environment."[73]

Principles include creating environments that welcome patients, families, and friends; valuing human beings over technology; and fostering a connection to nature and beauty.

A new building does not have to be built to adopt these principles. One hospital I worked at was ancient. In the washrooms, there were bulletin boards with infection control posters tacked on them.

I bought a little book of tear-off inspirational quotes. I started secretly putting up the quotes in the washrooms. I'd take them down and replace them randomly every few days. This subversive little project pleased me.

A mom who regularly brought her child to the hospital mentioned to the receptionist: "I always check in that bathroom to see if the quote has changed! It brings a smile to my face."

This does not have to be complicated.

I dug up funding for benches to be placed on a rooftop patio at one hospital. Another hospital embarked on a white board project. Installing white boards in patient room is not an aesthetic project – white boards have been shown to improve communication between staff and patients.[74]

Instead of complicated wayfinding signs or colours on the floor, one facility employed greeters at each entrance and encouraged staff to help people who were lost in their hallways.

Patients can be involved in renovation work too. At one hospital, pre-COVID, a patient suggested having a separate area for folks who were clearly sneezing or coughing to sit further away from others in Emergency. She offered another great idea: for each waiting room chair to have access to an electrical outlet to plug in phones. This was not only for convenience; it was for communication reasons, so patients could keep phones charged in order to be in touch with loved ones.

Another adjustment came in Day Surgery, where patients asked if there could be a private area for the surgeons to talk to loved ones after surgery. Previous to that, doctors would come out into the waiting room to give an update. There was no privacy for that conversation, which was overheard by all the other people sitting in the room.

This meant that the regular routine for the surgeons had to change. Instead of walking out to the waiting room, they had to call the names of the loved ones and meet them in an adjacent private room. This adjustment of the clinicians' flow was not minor – it took encouragement to get all the doctors on-board with the new routine. Slowly they saw the benefit of that privacy, so they could speak openly to families. This change lessened the anxiety of the other folks in the waiting room and saved them from the discomfort of overhearing a confidential conversation.

Involving patients with design makes sense. After all, they are the users of much of the space in a health care setting. Another advantage is that patients get an insight into staff struggles with space too. One mom, Tiffany Keiller, was involved with a PICU renovation at a children's hospital. Initially she thought that the family waiting area should be put in a room with an outside window. The staff person involved with the design suggested that the room with the window be the staff's break room instead. A thoughtful conversation ensued. Tiffany realized that staff spend more time in their break room than families do in the waiting room, and a consensus was reached that it was the staff who most benefitted from the room with the window.

My own mammogram clinic features muted lighting and soft classical music to set anxious patients at ease. These touches are small things done with care.

Engaging patients doesn't have to be 'us versus them' – patients demanding, staff yielding. It can be about mutual respect and understanding instead.

CHIPPING AWAY AT CHANGE

In my tenure at one children's hospital, I saw the beginnings of a culture shift. The managers embraced the notion of patient and family-centred care. I could see them light up when it happened – being connected with families helped them rekindle their initial passion for health care, which spreadsheets, HR policies, and Lean events worked to extinguish.

I knew I would have success if all staff had the confidence to partner with families who had previously been considered 'difficult.' This comes from a reframing if you realize there is no such thing as a difficult patient, only difficult situations.

Once I was at my desk and a receptionist ran in, breathless. 'There's a mom crying in the cafeteria,' she said. 'Please come and talk to her.'

Of course, I did. I sat down with this mom, who was distraught over the way the diagnosis for her child had been delivered. I stayed until she stopped crying. At the end, I gave her a hug and walked with her to her car in the parking lot.

Success would have looked like this: instead of running to me as the 'family person,' all staff would have the confidence and skills to sit down with a crying mom – and then I would have been happily out of a job.

I now had a full toolkit of strategies to softly encourage this revolution, to reignite passion in health care. I shared my own family stories, stood up before hospital audiences during a talk about complaints, announcing that I was a 'difficult mom' and showing my zombie mom picture (of me, complete with no bra, frizzy hair, slippers, and yoga pants) – trying to explain what it *feels* like to have a child in the hospital.

My assertion is that nothing changes until someone feels

something.

This tactic of vulnerability worked sometimes, but I was not for everybody. I'd be in meetings where the participants clearly thought I was off my rocker, showing PowerPoints with quotes and photos and communicating in stories instead of numbers or data. But I kept meeting with families, holding space for their stories, and bringing them back to staff. Once a therapist who had previously never spoken to me before – or even acknowledged my presence when we passed in the hall – came up to me after a talk.

'You really made me think about how I avoid families who are angry,' she said. 'Now I understand why they were angry.' This was a little light to encourage me to continue on.

Another clinician admitted: 'There's been a voice mail on my phone that I've been avoiding for a week. It is from a mom who has a complaint. I'm going to call her back right now.' Another lightbulb, another small win.

Giving staff choice and a voice in change helps, as does being dogged in your vision.

Many hospitals throw their hands up at the gargantuan task of engaging patients and improving their experience, but you can only do one thing at a time.

Start with that one thing. Then move onto the next thing. Repeat.

STAY CURIOUS, RESEARCHERS

Patient engagement does not only happen at the point of care or at the administrative level. Health researchers have been pioneers in engaging patients beyond people merely being research subjects. The best thing about researchers is that they ask questions and then listen carefully for the answer. This ability to be curious is what fuels innovation.

Why should patients lend their wisdom to researchers? It can be both selfish and altruistic. With every telling of our stories, there is learning – for both the storytellers and the listeners. If the research sees the light of day, it might just make a difference to future generations of patients. That's meaningful stuff.

I've been involved in dozens of research projects, but it is disheartening how often I was asked to be a partner only so I could write a letter for a grant proposal. I'd write words of support and then hear nothing back.

At a child health research conference, I was allotted five minutes out of a six-hour meeting to present the family perspective. I spoke fast, used an engaging illustration in my PowerPoint, but really? There needs to be more time assigned to understanding the experience of the actual people being researched.

At another research meeting, there was a roundtable of introductions, where everybody else introduced themselves by their academic credentials. By the time it was my turn, I squeaked out a joke about my pithy B.A. in English. These settings are intimidating to those patients who don't have a PhD.

I was at yet another research meeting at a small table discussion where I suggested the idea of peer support. The academic sitting beside me informed me that peers could never do this work – it would have to be a professional. That popped my balloon. After a while, my head hung down and I started to inspect my fingers. It was clear that they were in charge, I was there only to occupy a space, to check their boxes, and nobody was interested in hearing any wisdom from families to inform their work.

The main question is this: Did the research really make a difference in patients' lives? Is the intention behind the research to pad a researcher's CV or to make a positive difference in health policy or practice?

Researchers love toolkits, and there are many out there for partnering with patients in research.[75, 76]

Here is a layperson translation of the toolkits: Engage the subjects of your research early to make sure you are asking the right questions. Even better, do not think of them as subjects; consider them human beings.

Do not ignore those people you label 'hard to reach.' People are hard to reach because you aren't trying hard enough to reach them. Be creative and go to the people. This includes people with intellectual disabilities, who are often left out of research. Keep asking the questions to those who feel invisible in the system, erased by governments and minimized by media.

Do not assume that a patient organization speaks for all patients. They may tell you that they do but that's just not true. It is best to go to real people.

Ensure those you research don't feel used – let them know what ends up happening with the work and where it will be published.

Share stories and data in knowledge translation. If you touch hearts, you will change minds. Lean on the humanities to insert your own humanity into your reports and your presentations. Using infographics, photos, and quotes can help get your message across.

There is hope that the right research questions will eventually spark change in the health care world. The 'It Doesn't Have to

Hurt' campaign is a great example of this. Research about needle pain in children has seen the light of day because Dr. Christine Chambers partnered with influential parenting organizations to communicate practical suggestions about minimizing pain.[77]

This is where the future is: partnering with patients and families will help get research out of academic journals and into hands of the people who need it.

 This is as simple as adding a line in your budget to compensate patients to review research questions or inviting patients to be on an editorial board as the Journal of Family Nursing has done. The Journal of Medical Imaging and Radiation Sciences accepts narrative submissions from patients and health professionals.[78, 79]

One baby step at a time. One step, then another, then another. Change is within your control, including in the world of research.

REFRAMING COMPLAINTS

I f I was given the power to change one thing in health care, it would be how organizations receive feedback on patient experiences.

In an ideal world, patient feedback would be welcomed and embraced. All feedback would be seen as a gift.

Safe spaces would be created for feedback to be shared both at the point of care and within an organization. Patient relations departments would be staffed by peer workers and would be closely aligned with Quality Improvement initiatives. There would be an anonymous, online way to share stories of experiences. This information would then be given to hospitals so they could respond and improve. Managers would leave the hospital to go out to see patients in their own homes who had concerns.

Staff would also be able to speak up with their own opinions without fear of reprisal.

Complaints would be even encouraged and reframed as constructive feedback. Positive feedback would be shared directly with the staff member involved and their manager. Patients would hear about what changes were made, so they knew their time and effort mattered.

This is not a pipe dream. Recalibrating patient feedback policies and processes is within reach. Read on.

WHAT IS COUNTED, COUNTS

In the mid-1990's, I worked for the Health Department on a costing project. This project was based on the premise that patients with certain diagnoses in the hospital cost the system X amount of dollars. If someone had a heart attack, on average, the hospital would have to fund nursing staffing costs, diagnostic imaging, and medication. The complicated formula even considered the smaller resources, like food or cleaning services.

At the time, I jokingly called this 'The Counting Tissues Project' – in my mind, the value of a patient to a hospital was based on how many tissues they used. Now, as a patient, I don't find this funny. I am worth more than a box of tissues.

This approach to funding is flawed, yet our governments and health organizations continue to count the wrong things. Things have gone awry when patients are only considered as consumers of resources. I introduced the notion of counting the right things in *Bird's Eye View*.

> *"This means that the notion of "what counts is counted" would need to be adjusted. Listening would count. Holding someone's hand would count. Offering a hug would count. Care would be administered human being to human being, not professional to patient. For once we break down the walls between roles and acknowledge that we are all human, well, that's the place where compassion is born."* [80]

It is within a manager's control to count the activities of caring, not just consumption. Anyone in health care who supervises others can make caring their number one priority: the RN who is a preceptor for a student nurse, the unit clerk who is training a new staff member, the housekeeper who says hello to the patient before cleaning their room.

Organizations must consider valuing staff who make the time to connect with patients, instead of valuing only those who are efficient. This measurement would be possible when you track the patient experience.

Measuring the patient experience has been haphazard, especially in Canada. Patients might receive a survey at the end of their visit or stay. It is time to think beyond this old stale method of an inconsistently-distributed written survey to collect feedback.

 There are many steps to creating a feedback mechanism that isn't meaningless: involving patients in crafting the questions; giving many different options to answer the survey, like by paper, phone, web-based, or in-person. **Also key: allowing anonymous submissions, sharing the results back with the respondents, and ensuring there is action and change based on what is learned from the feedback.**

For more information, the Patient Experience Library has curated several studies that address connecting patient feedback with real world improvements.[81]

First, there needs to be safe spaces where people feel like they can give feedback without being punished. Many times, families in the children's hospital would tell me: "I don't want to say anything to that nurse/doctor/therapist because I'm afraid it would affect my child's care." The sad thing is, I couldn't reassure them that their child's care wouldn't be compromised if feedback was shared.

Not feeling safe to share feedback is a big patient safety and patient experience problem.

 One hospital hired peer support workers to go room to room to collect feedback from patients. Patients might feel more comfortable sharing with a peer rather than a staff member.

 Another children's hospital unit manager did rounds every day, to check on each family. The advantage to that is that the manager was able to influence policy change based on what she heard. She also demonstrated to the families that she cared about them and their children.

The best example of creating spaces online to give feedback is Care Opinion. The non-profit organization Care Opinion was founded in the UK and has spread to Scotland, Ireland, and Australia.

Dr. James Munro is their Chief Executive. He attests, "If we want healthcare cultures in which the experiences of people who use services matter, and lead to learning and change, then we must ensure those experiences are seen and heard within our healthcare settings."[82]

Care Opinion's mandate is to create safe environments for patients to share their stories online and to see other people's stories too.[83]

The simplicity of Care Opinion is what makes it brilliant. Patients share stories anonymously and the moderators give the feedback directly to the health organizations that delivered the care. Staff can respond to the feedback and use that information to improve the quality of their services. Care Opinion stories can be used for teaching as well as quality improvement.[84]

Anaesthesiologist Dr. Alika Lafontaine and his brother, dentist Dr. Kamea Lafontaine, created Safespaces Network for Indigenous patients to report their experiences. Safespaces collects the data and reports it on a map so patients know what health facilities to avoid because of reports of racism or inequitable care.[85]

Stories are how patients share their experiences. As Don Berwick says, "Person-centredness is not an element of an agenda for improvement, it is a precondition of improvement."[86]

If you don't ask the patients directly, you will never know how you are doing. You cannot have improvement unless you understand the patient experience. Improving quality and patient experience go hand in hand. It starts with asking the right questions and giving patients the ability to freely tell you what is important to them.

It is as crucial to consider what questions are asked in order to understand what can be done with the answers. The Sinclair Compassion Questionnaire is an example of a tool developed to measure compassion in health care by a researcher at the University of Calgary.[87]

There are other tools that collect patient feedback, like the Schwartz Center Compassionate Care Scale and the Picker Patient Experience Questionnaire.[88, 89]

Remember that all the tools in the world are a waste of time if positive change doesn't happen from the information collected. If patients bare their souls by sharing their stories with you and nothing is done with it, this is tokenism at its very worst.

YOU CAN'T HANDLE THE TRUTH

Like many patients, my attempts at giving feedback have been dismissed, rebuffed, and minimized. Emails have been ignored, I've been 'handled' or 'dealt with' and shown the door. The patient relations department's processes to escalate are often so complicated that I've just given up.

Plus, where I live, there is no independent body that investigates patient complaints. Health care does its own investigation, which is the ultimate conflict of interest: hospitals investigating themselves. If patients speak up in the media, hospitals refuse to respond, citing confidentiality.

Me squawking about patient experience feedback, even with simple requests like 'please turn off the blaring television in the waiting room' is nothing compared to the consequences of not listening to patients at the point of care in life-threatening positions.

However, it does beg the question – if you can't accept my feedback about the minor issues, how are you working with patients who have serious concerns that can lead to fatal consequences?

As Simon Sinek says, "Trust is built on telling the truth, not telling people what they want to hear."

In September 2020, a woman named Joyce Echaquan died in a Quebec hospital after her pleas for care from hospital staff were ignored and, horrifically, met with racism. Joyce videoed her experience on her phone, which is how we know her story. People are bravely coming forward to share their stories, and sometimes the media picks up on them for all to see these awful secrets in health care. [90, 91]

Racism is entrenched in health care. Health care systems have been built by and for white, affluent, able-bodied administrators. There can be fatal consequences to not believing patients. It is the ultimate betrayal when the people you go to for care actually don't care about you at all.

The late patient advocate Erin Gilmer clearly describes the concept of betrayal trauma in her blog, *Healthcare as a Human Right*.

> *"Others feel they have nowhere to go to speak up and are left feeling isolated in their pain. As such, betrayal trauma is left unaddressed and festers like an untreated wound."[92]*

Are patients who speak up in social media belittled or ignored? Are individual clinicians open to all feedback, without being defensive?

Do staff participate in reflective practice sessions when things go wrong? Do people say they are sorry?

Specific to Joyce Echaquan's heinous experience, I'll add these hard questions: Do staff value all people? Are some staff inherently racist?

Are staff allowed to be wrong? Are patients allowed to be right? Do other hospital staff speak up when they see something wrong?

These are difficult questions that need to be answered. One solution is for all feedback to be encouraged and welcomed, and for that feedback to be fed back into a Quality Improvement loop, which in turn will create better care.

It took six months of working at a children's hospital for me to differentiate between what people said was going on and what was really going on. Staff proudly told me they were family-centred, but slowly I built relationships with families and saw a different perspective. As I listened to families' experiences in the hospital, one issue repeatedly came up.

Families did not feel heard at the point of care. They did not feel safe in giving feedback about what was truly happening, for fear their child's care would be compromised. Often, they just swallowed this feeling, but sometimes they brought it forward through formal channels. They left voicemails or talked to unit managers, filled out pre-determined surveys, or followed the directions in the Patient Relations pamphlet handed to them if they had struggles with their child's care. Most of this didn't help.

If anybody responded to their voicemail messages, it was weeks later, when things began to fester even more. Staff avoided eye contact in the hall if families spoke to the unit manager. There was no feedback loop from surveys about what had changed for the better. Patient Relations departments – don't forget that these departments are part of the hospital – seemed more interested in protecting the hospital's interests than listening to and acting on family feedback. Even worse, the experience of being churned through a complaint process led to more trauma.

In short, the complaint system was terribly broken.

Organizations need to reframe the entire concept of complaints. Patients offering feedback is a gift.

The article "Caring for Care" published in the *Social Science and Medical Journal* describes feedback as:

> *"Vital to this was the premise that providing feedback was an enactment of care – care for other patients, certainly, but also care for healthcare as such and even for healthcare professionals."* [93]

If feedback is health care improvement, it will become an embedded part of the system. There are many reasons that patients offer feedback.

> *"[Patients offer feedback] to bring about changes to their care; to resolve an on-going issue; to raise concerns about care quality; to suggest*

*improvements; to express alarm, frustration or
even anger about the care received. They also used
online feedback to highlight good practice and to
thank, praise and acknowledge healthcare services
and staff."* [93]

The revolution begins with reframing feedback as being a vital part of health care. Health care must admit that it has a problem; that people who work in health care are real human beings who make mistakes. The God Complex needs to be abolished.

The reluctance to accept constructive feedback is prominent even in pediatrics and cancer services. They recoil from any feedback deemed as negative, in order to maintain their image of perfection. This is because these sectors heavily rely on fundraising to supplement their operational funds, and a perfect image certainly helps with raising those funds.

Fundraising stories of: "I'm cured and better than ever" might raise money, but they do not reflect the reality. Children die in children's hospitals. People die of cancer. Patients and families who do not embrace this false cheerleading narrative are quickly minimized, dismissed, and labelled as difficult.

What are complaints except for stories of things gone awry? Things go awry in health care. Patients know it and clinicians know it too. Making space for storytelling means making space for negative experiences too.

Looking at it from a purely system-centred point of view, there is value in the complaints. Respectfully encouraging all kinds of feedback at all levels in the organization also is the right thing to do from a patient safety and patient-centred perspective.

I do not like the word complaint. The word has an instant negative connotation. Complaints make people defensive. Couple that with health care training that teaches health professionals they must always be perfect – complaints don't fit into that narrative. If someone suggests that things aren't perfect after all, that rubs against the culture of perfection.

People who work in organizations must first admit that health care isn't perfect.

I think of complaints as constructive feedback. The way that staff and managers handle feedback – either at the point of care or in the organization – is a good indicator to determine if the culture is patient and family friendly.

Everything here applies to complaints from staff too. How do managers and human resources respond to staff feedback? Do they bury it? Smile tightly, fill out a form while nothing changes, except the feedback-giver is blacklisted?

The way in which staff feedback is welcomed is a feature of the internal culture of the organization.

Health care loves positive feedback. They use it for fundraising campaigns like radiothons, galas, and billboards. The story they make up about themselves as saviours is fed by glowing positive feedback, not concerns.

In the pivotal book *The Wounded Storyteller*, Arthur Frank explains health care's preference for restitution stories.[94] Restitution stories are positive ones, "the patients' stories tell what their treatments were, but the emphasis is on life after treatment: returning to I'm fine!"

Restitution stories do not tell what the actual experience is like in health care. What if things aren't fine?

There is no room for constructive feedback in these types of stories, only cheerleading. These stories are great for fundraising billboards, but not so good in depicting the nuances of health care, which do include the full gamut of the human experience.

My son with Down syndrome is an actor and has taken several

improv acting workshops. Improv hinges on relationships and the actors saying 'yes' to each other as they perform. If an improv actor said 'no' to a suggestion from another actor, the scene would just fizzle out.

The Alan Alda Center for Communicating Science leans on improv techniques to train scientists and clinicians.[95]

"Improvisation teaches scientists to become habituated to listening, and opening up to another person," explains Alda.[96]

What if feedback was met with curiosity and the attitude of: 'yes, and?' Instead of 'no, shut up, go away' and, by implication, 'quit being so hysterical.'

Listening and acting on patient feedback can only make health service and care better. For all the talk about quality improvement and health care transformation, do people in health care really want to change? That's a million-dollar question.

THE GOOD, THE BAD AND THE UGLY

The philosophy of creating a listening space for concerns can be a challenging concept for those who are used to fixing problems. Some problems are not to be fixed. They are meant to be listened to.

There are concerns that need practical solutions, like addressing a complaint of a dirty hospital bathroom, having stern conversations with rude staff, and working on lessening oppressive wait lists.

What if we tried to prevent concerns from happening? Oddly, health care talks a lot about prevention, but it is built to be reactive. So much time and grief would be saved if the experience was positive to begin with, therefore preventing concerns. If this isn't possible, the next step is to examine how concerns are handled. Are they ignored and buried? Many patients will say yes, this is what health organizations do.

I once got up in front of an audience of clinicians and announced: *I am a difficult mom.* I added, *if your child was hospitalized, you'd be a difficult mom too.*

I was on a mission to change the way family 'complaints' were viewed at this children's hospital.

My assertion was this: What if family complaints were seen as constructive feedback? What if staff sought out this feedback and saw complaints as wisdom? And then we applied that wisdom from patients and families that grew from difficult situations to improving the quality of care at the hospital? This would be a common-sense, but revolutionary notion.

In my work, I drew a process chart with a narrative to encourage a standardized way for staff and managers to respond to constructive feedback. I suggested that all staff – including those in clerical positions – be offered conflict management training to prevent issues from escalating. This type of training teaches things like saying yes instead of no and customer service concepts. While the term customer makes many folks shudder, think about if those who work in health care were committed to care and service. Drop the word customer and then you can simply think about serving patients and families instead.

A 'teach someone to fish' philosophy means that all staff are taught how to prevent conflict and how to handle it when it comes up, instead of immediately referring people to the patient relations department.

But first, I had to share my story about how I've been a difficult mom in an auditorium packed with hospital staff. As with most of my talks, my intention was for the staff to see themselves reflected in my words. I asked them to think about how they would respond if *they* had a concern when their loved one was in the hospital. I can't imagine that most health professionals would be meek and compliant family members.

I explained how it felt to be a mom in the hospital: *You may well be catching families when they are at a low point in their grief. I once had a wise physician tell me she teaches medical students that anger is often masking fear. Often anger is misdirected. Families may be seeking a diagnosis, reeling from a catastrophic accident, or are worn down by the system.*

I talked about the reasons why families can be challenging partners, like loss of control, fear, pain, grief, information overload, hopelessness, and cultural differences with staff. These things lead to staff assumptions and miscommunication – and a real fear of negatively affecting their child's care if they speak up.

That's a lot to grapple with.

Certain practical things can make it worse. Lack of sleep. No coffee. Being hungry. Worry about other kids at home. Anxiety about money and work. Compound that with stress about their beloved child-patient and you create a *difficult situation, not a difficult family,* says an article called "Difficult Families."[97]

In my talk I gently suggested that people please pause and always consider how families are feeling. You might not be able to put yourself in their shoes, but you can move towards a kinder understanding of their perspective. One lesson I have learned from life is 'don't poke the bear.' Why make angry people angrier? There is no healing in that.

I had been introduced to many families at the hospital during their complaint process. I didn't want to be the complaint lady – instead, I wanted to teach staff how to prevent complaints and the way to do that is by being patient and family-centred. I suggested how to respond to negative feedback when it inevitably occurs.

I think we can all agree that hospitals are not perfect places. Immediately shuffling people off to some complaint lady only minimizes their concerns, absolves staff of any responsibility, and teaches folks nothing.

The staff just didn't know what to do with these families. They felt defensive and took negative feedback personally. This is human nature. Some wrote families off as 'difficult' or 'hysterical,' which is an easy way to stereotype and dehumanize people so you don't have to think of them as people anymore. It is good to notice if we are categorizing people and why.

All families and patients have constructive feedback after an experience. Health care just needs to be brave enough to ask them.

When I became a breast cancer patient, I had a lot of feedback for the cancer hospital. None of it has ever been considered or implemented. I filled out surveys, met with a manager, asked to meet with the VP of Patient Experience (and was ignored), wrote on my blog, appeared on major health care podcasts, and finally wrote a book about my perspective as a breast cancer patient.

The cancer hospital has consistently ignored, minimized, and dismissed me over the years.

It is up to those working in systems to honour all voices, not just the positive ones. You can't be heroes all of the time, but every single person who works in health care can be a healer. Please help us heal. Don't turn away from our suffering. You will learn something from what we have to say.

Author Donna Thomson wrote about the family from hell from her point of view as a caregiver. "All this talk of difficult families got me thinking just how, when the going gets the toughest, we are demonized by those working for systems that cannot meet our escalating needs."[98]

Delaying response to a concern makes it even worse, and layers yet another concern on top of the original one: lack of responsiveness. Then there are two concerns, not just one.

 Vow to have a standard response time to patient and family concerns. Pick up the phone. Arrange an in-person meeting. Any response can help de-escalate the situation and prevent further misunderstandings.

Patients and families who have experienced adverse events have the most valuable of all feedback to share. It is in fact an honour for health organizations to have patients approach them with their stories. The wisdom generated from when things go wrong is very powerful. Patients and families are driven to influence change, so the event doesn't happen to anybody else. This gives some meaning to often traumatic and sad situations.

Some of the best patient council members are those who found their way to the boardroom table through a concern or an adverse event. Do not be afraid of these patients and families, as they can help you with your work.

But in order to be open to learning from these concerns, one must learn humility. Hospital culture must allow for mistakes, make them visible and transparent, and support their staff to respond to errors in a respectful way.

Don't push people away and squash their voices. That makes it worse. Say yes instead of no as much as possible. Say you are sorry that this has happened. This does not assign blame to you, it merely expresses regret for something that has occurred. The power of a genuine apology is strong. Listen.

Pause and think – how would I feel if it was me?

Patients who are offering up feedback can help you in your work. From experience, I know best how to explain blood draws to my son or how to comfort him when he's upset. We can help professionals if only we work together as a team, for we each have our own unique expertise to bring to the bedside. Remembering that we are all on the same team will only benefit the patient in the end.

At one children's hospital, I was proud of every single one of the four patient care managers because they traveled with me to meet with families outside of the hospital. A manager of a clinic drove with me twice to a coffee spot in a family's neighbourhood – an hour away from the hospital – to meet with a group of moms who had feedback about the clinic's service. That could not have been easy for the manager to do, as much of the feedback would be considered constructive, not complimentary. The manager did the hard thing. Afterwards, the families she met helped her review survey questions for other families in the clinic. A relationship was formed.

Another manager and I met a mom in the shared area of her condo. There was a meeting with a manager and a mom in a local coffee shop. Yet another manager and I drove to a distant city to meet a mom for lunch in her hometown.

At one meeting about an adverse event, the mom and dad weren't able to leave the hospital, so I asked what outside food they had a craving for. I picked up sushi and brought it back to the meeting. All of us sharing a meal together made for a friendlier meeting.

The important thing was that these meetings were not one-offs. The managers followed up with the families about what action had happened because of their feedback. Relationships were formed and loops were closed, which made the time spent together meaningful.

Feedback of any kind is a gift.

PHILOSOPHY FOR STAFF WORKING WITH PEOPLE WHO HAVE CONCERNS

Here are practical suggestions about working with patients and families who have feedback.

1. Check in with how you are feeling. Don't judge your feelings but be aware of them. Take some deep breaths. If you can, go for a walk before you pick up the phone or meet with people.

2. Don't delay responding. Delays make things fester.

3. Avoid escalations over email. Be respectful and suggest meeting in person if possible (see #7).

4. Consider framing complaints as constructive feedback and be open to learning in order to be better – both personally and professionally. We can all improve.

5. Consider how constructive feedback can feed into quality improvement activities to improve the experience for future patients and families.

6. I have found that the root of 90% of concerns was that people didn't feel listened to, so...

7. Start by setting a warm tone for authentic listening. Consider meeting outside the hospital, going to the families in their own communities – at their homes or a local coffee shop. Give families choice in when and where they would like to meet. Don't drag them into the hospital again.

8. Suspend the notion of being a fixer and show up as a healer instead.

9. Be okay with saying "I'm sorry."

10. Be okay with saying "I don't know."

11. Ask the family what they'd like to see as a solution.

12. Follow up and do the things you promise to do.

13. Consider asking the patients or families if they'd like to share their wisdom with others in some way. In my experience, in time, those with concerns have the most valuable lessons to teach to Grand Rounds, medical students, committees, and councils (if they so want). Many people have a strong need to improve situations in the system so that they don't happen to others too.

14. Take care of yourself after challenging situations at work. Engage in reflective practice techniques, think about how things went and how you would make them better next time. Do not forget to be kind to yourself too.

NURTURE THE HUMANITIES

In 1987, I transferred from a nursing program to the Faculty of Arts. I was supposed to be a nurse, but I left after completing half my degree. Instead, I graduated with a Bachelor of Arts (B.A.) in English, with concentrations in Shakespeare and art history.

As an odd duck, I remained in health care with my English degree. In the 1980's, the decade of yuppies and rampant capitalism, anybody with a liberal arts degree was mocked as an artsy-fartsy. But I embraced my degree along with my two years of nursing. My arts degree gave me a broad perspective, a love of reading, and the ability to see different points of view. For me, nursing was not like that – it was very black and white, with little patience for the grey in-between.

The trouble with the black and white view is that while clinical tasks mostly fell neatly in tidy boxes, human beings do not.

My first job with my fresh B.A. was as a Staffing Coordinator in a hospital. I called nurses at 6 am, asking if they'd come into work. What does this have to do with Shakespeare? Not much, except I had to build relationships with the nurses in the float pool, and I did that through chit-chat, being curious about their lives and what mattered to them. These were not 'hard' scientific skills; they were the 'soft' skills that I had learned from attending seminars and reading books.

I remained in health care but never became a clinician. Years later, I had the personal experiences of giving birth to a baby with Down syndrome and then later, being diagnosed with breast cancer. I began to realize that there was power in the humanities, like stories, art, and music, to help people heal.

The humanities in health care are often referred to as medical humanities. We must cast a wider net than only medicine, for health care is more than medicine. It is not just physicians who benefit from the sensitivity and open-minded thinking that the humanities encourage. Most of the references that you will find are from the genre of medical humanities, but we must apply them to broader health care situations.

Medical schools are coming around to the idea that including the humanities can improve education. An article from a Greek medical journal says, "Medical humanities provide insight into human conditions, illness and suffering, perception of oneself, as well as into professionalism and responsibilities to self and others; colleagues and patients."[99]

The humanities help in all areas of health care: nursing, rehabilitation medicine, administration, clerical staff – and don't forget – patients and families.

Stories, art and music are useful tools for many things. First, to create healing environments. Think of the last waiting room you saw. Was it a jarring or a healing environment? Was it a row of hard chairs, bright lighting, haphazard signs on the wall, the noise of a television? Or was it comfy, with accessible seating, soft lights, welcoming signage, and quiet music?

There are many ways to harness the humanities to create gentler environments for all – through photographs, music, dance, plays, books, humour or visual art.

Having safe spaces to share stories is useful for reflective practice for staff. Stories shared by patients and families can be harnessed for healing and advocacy. Stories can motivate, inspire, and educate.

Stories can be expressed beyond the written and spoken word, through genres like photography, music, or the visual arts, but let's start with words. Stories are simply the way human beings talk about what happened to them.

There are benefits in talking about – and listening to – wisdom that comes from the suffering and the healing.

TELLING OUR UNTOLD STORIES

There are many terms for stories in health care: case studies, medical histories, narratives, and experiences. Stories are the way that patients talk about their experiences. We all have a story to tell, if only there was someone to listen.

There is evidence that stories are important tools for education. I'm not out to prove the power of stories but think of the last time you read a book, watched television, or went to a movie. As human beings, we are all drawn to stories.

Don Berwick, from his book *Promising Care* writes:

> *"Radical transformation was not possible until
> we looked at the people we want to help, and we
> see ourselves; when we realize that their needs out
> there, are our needs, in here...the moats we dig
> between patients and clinicians can drain spirit
> from both."* [100]

We can fill in these moats by sharing our respective stories.

"The phrase "soft evidence" is also used to distinguish patient feedback from the "hard evidence" of statistics," says the Patient Experience Library. [101]

Being a soft person myself, I don't think there is anything wrong with soft. I'd rather sleep on a soft pillow than a hard floor. However, the words soft, anecdotal, qualitative, and stories are not respected in health care. The soft is dismissed for the hard.

 Think of a story about health care that made an impact on you. It could be a patient story, or a story in the media. *The Big Sick* film, *SickBoy* podcast, Karen Klak's *Happy Faces Only* book, and Heather Lanier's *Good*

and Bad Are Incomplete Stories We Tell Ourselves TED Talk are examples of health stories.[102, 103, 104, 105]

The pandemic has ensured that health care is in the media all the time. Pre-COVID, internal communications people made sure that health care stories never hit the front page of the newspaper. With the pandemic and the Internet, that stream is 24/7. The pandemic has shown the whole world knows how all-consuming health care can be.

What is missing from the Public Health Officers' speaking notes are stories. People with COVID are referred to as cases. People who have died of COVID are deaths.

Human beings have been distilled down to numbers because you don't feel anything for numbers. This is a purposeful public relations tactic. It is meant to dehumanize the suffering of the pandemic. Not talking about people who have gotten COVID nor people who have died from COVID literally depersonalizes them. They are numbers and not people anymore.

Humanity in health care must be reclaimed. As Audre Lorde says, "Your silence will not protect you." [106]

The way we break the silence is by telling our stories.

DO NO HARM

Safe places must be built to share stories. Both the organizers and the audience have responsibilities when someone shares their health care tales – whether it is a patient, family, or staff member.

Being an organizer is more than just asking someone to show up and tell their story, without support or direction. Being an audience member is more than passively sitting in your chair while someone speaks.

> *When I see people stand fully in their truth...my gut reaction is what a bad ass. - Brené Brown*

I like to challenge organizers and audience members to think of a time when something painful happened to them. Then ask them to imagine what it would feel like to write a story about it, stand up on a stage in front of the very people who contributed to that painful time, and talk to them about it. Everybody deserves respect for opening up about difficult experiences, but I have a special place in my heart for those courageous enough to go public – by standing on a stage or behind a byline of a written story.

Therefore, stories have to be solicited and supported in a respectful way. There is harm to the storytellers and the audiences if storytelling opportunities go south. Audience members must commit to active listening and applying a take-away from the story to their own practice.

As Hawthornthwaite et al. writes in *The Permanente Journal* "...patient stories could serve as lessons or reminders about the dimensions of PFCC (patient and family-centred care) and could inspire changes to practice."[107]

This is one of the few studies that talks about audience responsibility. In this study, storytellers reported an immensely rewarding experience and highlighted the value of educating and connecting with participants. However, they said that the experience could also pose emotional challenges. This goes back to the bad ass storytellers. We must protect the bad asses.

One of the struggles for storytellers is that they rarely hear back if they made a difference.

I have had dozens of post-talk surveys shared with me – with both good and constructive feedback. My favourite good piece is this: *She changed the way I practiced medicine.* But the comment was anonymous, and I don't know what I said that influenced the audience member. I say a lot of things in hopes that something sticks. It would be good to know what sticks.

Once I had a social worker stop me in the hall a couple of weeks after a talk I did at a children's hospital. One of my main messages to folks who work with new families is to say congratulations instead of I'm sorry when a baby who has Down syndrome (or any unexpected diagnosis) is born. She told me that after she heard me speak, she'd try to say congratulations first to see what happened.

She said she now offers a joyful congratulations instead of sad condolences to families, and it reframes the whole relationship with families, to begin on a path based on strengths instead of pity. If you are an audience member and hear an idea from a speaker, why not try it out and see what happens?

Those who ask patients or staff to share their health care stories also need to lead the work of building the safe space.

First, think about your why. Why are you asking people to share their stories? Is it for inspirational reasons? To educate the audience? To be provocative to trigger reflection?

Tokenism is when you are ushered into the middle of a meeting to give a talk and then told to leave afterwards. It feels awful knowing you've just been used and disposed of.

Organizers must be clear with storytellers about the reason why they are asked to share their story. If the storyteller consents and is aligned with the why, then all is well. There are many patients and families who are fine with sharing their story for hospital fundraising reasons. This is fine as long as they are aware of the reason and do not feel coerced or obligated into sharing their stories.

The most important question for organizers is: Are you using stories or are you using people for their stories?

A BAZILLION STORIES

I have a bazillion tales about sharing my story in health care settings – some are good and some are bad. I learn a lesson with every speaking engagement.

Once I was the closing speaker at a nursing conference in a prairie city in the middle of winter. A blizzard started up when I was speaking and many of the nurses had driven in from rural areas. Even before I stopped talking, people started to evacuate the room to drive home before the roads got too bad. By the time I was done, there was nobody left. I was standing solo in an empty room.

Lesson? Well, you can't control the weather, but you can have someone assigned to say thank you to the speaker and escort them back to their car to say good-bye. The after-storytelling part matters.

Here is a story of the ole awkward 'middle of the meeting' talk. I was set to speak to a group of Neonatal Intensive Care Unit (NICU) doctors. I was supposed to arrive in the middle of a meeting and then leave afterwards. When I showed up, the room was packed and dark and there was nowhere for me to sit! An awkward musical chair session followed. Lesson: Save a chair for your speaker and make them feel welcomed, not like an intrusion.

Another time I spoke about patient and family-centred care to a group of dental professionals. The talk was on a Friday night, after work, to kick off a weekend conference. The audience was flat. I don't know if it was my content, or me, or the time of day, but I couldn't get them to crack a smile. One audience member even nodded off in the front row. There were no questions afterwards and everybody abruptly got up and left. Clearly, I had bombed. Evening sessions are brutal. Having a moderator to encourage the audience to ask questions would have helped.

I don't think audiences realize we can see them looking at their phones, chatting with their friends, and falling asleep. It is important to honour storytellers by listening attentively.

I had a talk in a fancy venue after my book was released. I'm the type of speaker who needs the comfort of paper speaking notes, even if I never refer to them. I'm a terrible memorizer.

The fancy stage had no podium for my notes. I was to wander around the stage holding a microphone. I began sweating when the organizers told me this when I showed up. The irony of being an experienced speaker is that I now have more confidence to ask for things than I would have a decade ago.

I need a table or podium, I said with a smile. That will ruin the look of the stage, they said. I stood there smiling and didn't say a word. Clearly, I was not budging. I got the podium. Organizers, check with speakers beforehand to see what accommodations they need.

On another stage, there were only bar stools for the panel members to be perched on. I do not like this new trend. Again, there was nowhere to put my paper – and I like to scribble notes during a panel so I can respond to other speakers – plus I was wearing a dress. It was precarious to balance on a little stool wearing a dress.

Sure enough, when I saw the pictures of the event afterwards, my dress was tucked up under the chair. Thank goodness it was a black dress and I was wearing black tights, so it wasn't my bare thigh hanging out for all to see.

I'm mortified even typing out this story. The lesson learned: equipment and set-up matter to storytellers.

Technology makes a difference too. I showed up to speak to a class of pharmacy doctoral students. Typically, the person who asked me to speak is there to introduce me and help me set up my presentation. There was nobody there to greet me. I couldn't find parking and had problems locating the room at the large university.

When I finally arrived, there was a class of students looking at me expectantly. I put my USB in their laptop. The projector didn't work. I started sweating. I was obviously struggling, but nobody helped me. They just stared at me. Finally, I asked, 'Can somebody help me?' and a young man got up reluctantly.

When my talk finally got started, most of the class had their head down, typing away at their keyboards. Were they on Facebook or taking notes? I couldn't tell. They obviously had not been prepared for my arrival as a patient speaker. I felt like a fool sharing my story with such an inattentive audience.

Worst of all, I was in the washroom after my talk. Some of the students came in and I could hear them talk about me when I was in the stall. They were saying that they don't have time to do "all this kindness stuff." Hot tip: Watch where you talk about the speaker because she could be in the washroom stall.

These stories all come with lessons about how audiences and organizers could have made the experience for the storyteller better.

They have to do with before (prep), during (support), and after (debrief and action).

Do the storytellers know the intention of the talk? Are they asked about what technical requirements and accommodations – like podiums, tables, microphones – they need to be successful?

Is parking clear and does someone meet them in a common place like a lobby to take them to the room? This is not demanding rock star stuff. These are supports to create safe environments for someone who is honouring you with their story.

Is the presentation pre-loaded and tested? Is there someone assigned to trouble-shoot technology? I've had two talks where the technology completely failed, there was no back up and I had to resort to having no visuals when I depend on pictures and quotes to complement my speaking notes.

Does someone introduce the storyteller beyond reading a biography? Do they let the audience know why the topic should be important to the group? Do they remind the audience of their responsibility to be respectful? And do they moderate the talk if contentious questions come up?

Afterwards, does someone say thank you so the storyteller isn't left awkwardly standing there? Walk them back to their car? Send a thank you note afterwards? Follow up to ensure the storyteller is paid and feedback is shared with them?

There is a lot to consider when asking people to share their stories. I hope this chapter doesn't scare you off. Inviting storytellers is well worth it. It can move the needle on system and individual change in health care. If you touch hearts, you might just change minds.

Never forget that it is an honour to bear witness to someone's story.

ON HECKLERS

Feeling confident that you have everything figured out? Life has a way of unexpectedly knocking you off your pedestal.

I've been heckled three times in my speaking career. Once was in 1995 when I was working for the Health Department and presenting a new funding formula to a physician group. The doctors were very angry about the new formula. I remember telling my co-presenter afterwards – gosh, I wish you had thrown your coat over me and escorted me off the stage. It was that bad.

The second time was over a decade ago. Another mom and I were presenting to genetics clinic staff about the value of peer support for parents who have a baby or baby-to-be with a new diagnosis of Down syndrome. We were showing photos of our kids, who were three and six at the time.

A geneticist got up in the back of the room and said, "What happens when your kids aren't so cute anymore?" Both of us speakers stood there, frozen and horrified. This was a man who disclosed prenatal diagnoses of Down syndrome to families. Afterwards, I wished I had retorted: "What happened to you when you weren't so cute anymore?" But alas, I don't think very quickly on my feet.

The third time I was heckled was in 2015. I flew to another city to speak at an Emergency Department conference. My messages were about kindness and compassion in health care, and how the little things matter to patients and families.

My talk was called "Seven things that mean a lot to patients." I talked about the stress of finding parking, and the anxiety associated with the Emergency waiting room, and the big stop sign that says STOP AND WASH YOUR HANDS that greets patients when they first walk in the door. I asked – why not try to provide a little comfort to patients so they aren't so stressed and angry when they arrive? Less agitated patients would benefit health professionals too.

My heckler took great issue with my thoughts on the stop sign. He felt that patients should be told to stop and wash their hands and that patients thought that the 'H' on hospitals meant hotel, and he didn't have time for that.

He went on and on about how awful patients were and now it is all a blur to me as I stood there swallowing back my tears. Other people chimed in about how demanding patients were and I realized, in horror, how awful the emergency experience must be for both patients and staff. One nurse actually said: I treat patients the way they treat me. If they are mean to me, I'm mean right back.

I had no response to this rising hostility. Like at my first heckling experience 20 years earlier, I needed a coat thrown over me and an escort off the stage, but nobody did. Finally, a young nurse put up her hand and was handed the microphone: "Thank you for your talk," she said quietly. "I learned some things that I could do better at work. I'm going to try to slow down and not rush so much." I croaked out a thank you to her, grateful for her bravery to speak up.

There are so many lessons here. Patient speakers are sharing their stories and allowing themselves to be vulnerable. Audience members, please respect that. Patient speakers, protect your hearts and be aware that things can go sideways. I had obviously forgotten that – the aggression that came at me felt like a slap. As a speaker, I needed to toughen myself to the fact that not everybody will agree with my message, and that's okay.

Organizers, please assess your audience carefully. If your audience is hostile to hearing the patient experience, perhaps consider waiting to invite a speaker until the environment is less adversarial.

Fear of conflict when you are standing up on a stage is why rational people shy away from public speaking. I generally speak to engaged audiences who are open to hearing about love and compassion. I've presented over 100 times since I've begun this work – so a few hecklers out of 100 isn't that bad.

I'm trying to make lemonade out of lemons. My experience onstage at this talk in 2015 knocked me right off my feet. I took a break from speaking engagements after this so I could draw my own boundaries with sharing my story. I reflected on the harm that can come to patients telling their stories in public places. I pondered the responsibility of the organizers and audiences to respectfully treat people who are brave enough to get up on stage.

My best wisdom usually comes from painful experiences, not the good ones.

SHARING THE PODIUM

Who gets to share their story? Whose stories are left out?

There are many ways to share the podium. Patients presenting with health professionals. Families presenting with youth. Patients presenting with patients. Think beyond the middle-aged, middle-class white ladies like me – think of people with diverse stories to provide a variety of life experiences. Stories should reflect the diversity of the people in the waiting room.

It was my job to work with family speakers at children's hospitals. I did not always do that well. It was easier to default to asking moms who were just like me. I amassed wisdom through my mistakes.

I was introduced to a woman who was the mom of a young child with a rare disease. She was interested in speaking to a group of nursing students.

My first mistake was assuming that she used email to communicate, like I did. It is important to ask people how they like to keep in touch. She preferred texting, not email or phoning – those were my ways of communicating, not hers.

Next, I asked her if she'd like to meet in a coffee shop close to her home. She hesitated. She said, "I usually don't meet in coffee shops," and I realized I had mis-stepped again. I had suggested a hipster coffee place that featured $6 cups of coffee. Not everybody can afford or wants to spend $6 on a drink like me. Also, a local shop by her home did not offer her privacy to share her story, did it? She might run into neighbours there and the setting wasn't exactly a safe place to share confidential information.

She invited me to her apartment after her workday ended. I had to be open enough to go to her home and have flexible work hours so I could meet at 6 pm. My employer had a policy that allowed me to visit someone's home (I had to tell a 'buddy' where I was). I figured out the logistics from my end and showed up at her door.

We had a good conversation around her kitchen table. Her boyfriend and son were at home so there was lots of chit-chat and it was an informal meeting. I had to suspend any idea of an agenda and go with the flow.

I said, "Do you want to have your own PowerPoint slides?" She was polite enough not to roll her eyes at me, "Um, PowerPoint isn't my thing. I don't have a laptop."

I tried again, "How would you like to talk to the students?" Silence. "Would you like to write a talk? You could read it?"

No, that wasn't okay either. We bantered back and forth for a few minutes. She didn't want to stand up in front of the classroom. I understood this.

"You could totally sit down on a chair on the stage," I said. She thought that would be okay. We still weren't sure about the content.

Finally, we decided together that I would interview her, and ask her questions in front of the audience. She was comfortable with that idea.

On the day of the talk, I met her near the bus stop and we walked together to the auditorium. We sat together and had a great chat about having a kid with a disability in front of the audience. The students loved her – she was natural and funny. I was there to help her shine.

Her idea about sitting down and just talking was a much more effective way to communicate than reading off bullets on a PowerPoint slide.

Afterwards, we went out for lunch together to debrief. I picked up the tab and gave her the honorarium we had agreed upon. I offered to drive her home instead of her taking the bus. "No, I'm good," she said and she was gone. Later, I shared the students' positive evaluation comments with her. It was the beginning of a relationship.

Lesson? Meet people where they are at – literally and figuratively. I've shared the podium with many people, including my son's community support worker. We presented to a group of physical education students at a university. I spoke with a pharmacist at a pharmacy association conference. I presented to a group of pediatric residents with a geneticist and another mom. I co-presented at Grand Rounds and Perinatal Grand Rounds with my son's pediatrician.

Memorably, the nurse coordinator for my son's clinic and I shared the podium at a conference in Washington. I spoke with two other authors of health care books at a hospital in Melbourne. My husband and I presented at the World Down Syndrome Congress in Dublin.

The wonderful thing about co-presenting – as opposed to just lecturing – is that you have the chance to work with someone beforehand to craft your talk.

Using a collaborative presentation model is often more powerful than having one person stand up and speak from their perspective. The patient plus professional model is a particularly clever one. It gives space for stories from diverse perspectives. Professionals who share both personal stories and research alongside patients are especially impactful. There's nothing like offering content to both the left-brained and the right-brained folks in the audience.

Co-presenting models partnerships between patients and professionals. I'm a layperson often speaking to a room full of highly educated and credentialed individuals. My B.A. in English doesn't go very far in that crowd. Having one of the audience's colleagues co-present with me helps to give me credibility, too. I wish it was enough to be 'just' a mom or cancer patient, but that's sadly not the reality. Being a layperson with a lifetime of experience should be enough but it's not. (Note: it is enough to me).

It also helps my co-presenter reflect on their own practice, and how they've made a difference in a patient's life, and what their own philosophies are about patient-centred care. My co-presenter to a group of pharmacy students told two fabulous stories about patient-centred care from when he was in pharmacy practice. One involved always helping patients lost in the hospital corridors, and the other was about understanding the patient perspective. I think having a mentor talk about his own experiences, including the challenges and rewards of delivering compassionate care was crucial. It helped make it real for the students.

At another conference, speaking with another pharmacist, my co-presenter poignantly shared his own story of supporting his wife in the hospital. You could hear a pin drop in the room. The audience of health professionals could see themselves reflected in his story more than they could see themselves reflected in mine. I don't take this personally. This is human nature, even though the work of the audience should also be to adapt take-aways from any kind of stories to their own practices.

A caution: ensure co-presenters are not only those who work in health care – for those folks might carry a lot of wisdom, but they are also privileged by their positions. It is crucial to offer the 'regular patient' perspective and not slide into the laziness of 'everybody is a patient' and only ask your colleagues to speak.

Having a co-presenter also makes me a better presenter. This ensures I don't become complacent and just talk from a canned script. I must work with my colleague to tailor words, and that's a good thing. I can run speaking notes past them and incorporate their suggestions. It is my Quality Assurance check (plus, everybody needs an editor or a fresh set of eyes on any kind of content). It keeps me on my toes. My co-presenter can also help me understand the audience and that makes me a better speaker.

Sharing the podium ensures that neither of us are dangling when we are asked questions, and we can help bail each other out if things get hard.

When a health professional enquires about me speaking, I often respond: "Will you present with me?" If not, that's okay too – but I meet with them to get an understanding of the audience, and what they want the key take-aways to be. I also ask: "What would you say if you were up there with me?" and use their wisdom to craft my words.

I've learned a lot over the past few years, standing on that stage and talking to an audience. My main lesson is that public speaking is about your audience; it isn't about you. I do whatever I can to supplement the message I'm trying to get across – and that can include sharing the limelight too.

STORIES AS HEALING

"The way out of the chaotic storm of illness is to tell stories."[108] I talk a lot about storytelling at the point of care in my first book. Do stories also heal patients when they are told on a stage with a microphone? Or are these stories only healing and educational for the audience?

The answer, as with all general questions directed at patients, is that it depends. How do you know when it is safe to tell your story?

Ironically, the more I experienced I am as a speaker, the more I am taken care of. There are prep meetings, debriefs, careful consideration of my technology and equipment requirements. Plenary speakers get treated more respectfully than those new to the public speaking arena, who need extra care to keep them going.

There is much written about 'using' stories to advance quality improvement projects, medical education, or health research in various academic journals.

> *"Telling the story of one patient's experience of care can memorably illustrate improvements or problems in a care pathway," says the Health Foundation in the UK.[109] An article in the Journal of Further and Higher Education states, "...patients' stories prepare students by allowing them to reflect on their practice in the safety of the academic environment."[110]*

From the British Medical Journal: "There is a growing trend to use storytelling as a research tool to extract information and/or as an intervention to effect change..." [111]

Note the words 'using' and 'extract.' There is much information about the benefits of patient storytelling for the audience, but there is scant research about the effect on the storytellers.

The Ottawa Hospital has created a tool for storytellers to gauge their readiness to tell their stories. "Patient storytellers are retelling or reliving their patient stories and, as such, run the risk of experiencing psychological trauma." [112]

Other research has looked at the role of emotion for patient storytellers.

"However, emotion remained unpredictable and had lingering implications for storytellers' vulnerability," says an article called *Beyond Catharsis: the nuanced emotion of patient storytellers in an educational role.*[113]

This is not to discourage organizations from engaging patient storytellers. It is a call to support your storytellers well. You don't need to wait for a research study to treat storytellers with respect and dignity, just as you would do at the bedside.

The classic book *The Wounded Storyteller* says, "Stories have to repair the damage that has been done to the ill person's sense of where she is in life, and where she may be going. Stories are a way of redrawing maps and finding new destinations."[114]

I have been guilty of sharing my story with whoever asks me: media, conference organizers, foundations, and health organizations. I did this for many different reasons: I was flattered to be asked; my voice had often been suppressed in clinical settings, so finally I had a chance to be heard; telling my story was healing; I felt pressure to speak up for those who couldn't; I wanted to use my story to make change in the world; I wanted to inspire others to be more compassionate and kind; I wanted to be liked; I am not (that) scared of public speaking; I felt obliged to give back to the organization that was asking.

I wasn't that choosy, and I mostly said yes, yes, and yes.

My suggestion for storytellers is to pause and think: Why am I telling my story? Is my intention for speaking in alignment with the organization asking me to present? Can they be trusted? Have they shown me respect? Is your Spidey sense tingling? Is your gut telling you something beyond just the regular anxiety that comes with speaking?

If these answers are 'I'm not sure' or 'no,' then it is best to decline.

Here's an easy assessment: is everybody else telling their story being paid to be there and you are not? Then for sure say no. That's just plain old inequity and that's not fair. Don't do paid work for free.

Do you feel ready to tell the hard parts of your story in a constructive way? After my cancer treatment was done, I was asked to share my cancer story at a conference. Upon reflection, I realized that I was still terribly angry about my experience in the hospital. I had not fully processed the medical and emotional trauma of having cancer. It would not have been healthy for me to stand up before an audience and share my story in public, so I said no.

Consider if you are a family member: are you sharing your own story as a caregiver or your loved one's story? If it is your loved one's story, is this your story to tell?

This pause to think about and assess requests is new for me. I still believe it is only through stories that we will change this world. I'll continue to share on my website, as this is a platform I can control. My quotes won't get taken out of context and I oversee my own headlines and messaging.

I vow to only engage with spaces that are safe to share my patient and family story. I will work only with organizers, interviewers, and audiences who recognize it is an honour to be given a glimpse into a patient or family's life and who behave accordingly.

If I sound jaded, please understand that this is hard-fought wisdom. Our stories are a version of ourselves. They are a gift. Don't give yourself away.

COACHING STORYTELLERS

Making space for people to tell their stories helps rekindle empathy. It reminds staff what is important to the people they serve.

What matters is sometimes surprising: someone who helps us when we are lost in the hall. It is the hand on our shoulder, the hug, the holding of the hand. It is the kind word, and the time spent sitting together in silence. It is being called by our first names instead of 'Mom' and our children being addressed directly and first in the clinic room. It is the knock on the door before you come in, the smile, the time to connect through eye contact.

Patients and families can tell you what's important to them if you give them a chance. Some organizations include patient stories at the beginning of all their management meetings. One of my workplaces began with: What did you learn from a patient or family recently? I've opened provincial meetings about child health with a story about why the system work they are doing makes a difference to families' lives. This can help ground the participants in why they are doing what they do.

Scheduling patient talks during existing staff time is an organic, natural way to include stories in regular sessions, as opposed to creating a special patient event.

This embeds stories where they belong – in all gatherings in health care, not just segregated ones. Whenever there is an existing talk, think: how can I include a story in this? This can be staff stories, as the realm of storytelling is not just restricted to patients. Orientation, staff meetings, rounds, professional development events, standing committees – these are all examples of where stories can appear.

There is real and important work involved with coaching and bringing in a patient or family speaker. It is impossible to have a 'real' patient speaker at every meeting, of course, but that shouldn't stop efforts to bring in this important voice. In-person is always preferred but think creatively about how the patient perspective can be shared. Perhaps it is via data through surveys, feedback forms, and case studies, or sharing results from interviews with patients. This may not be the pure patient story, but better to have some nod to the value of the patient perspective than none at all.

Written stories work too, as do patient videos. An easy way to create a video is to record and edit a Zoom call where a patient is having a conversation with an experienced interviewer.

It is supremely unfair to simply ask a patient to show up and tell their story. There are so many complex aspects of stories. Not setting an expectation of what the organizer is looking for in a story does not set the speaker (nor the audience) up for success. Public speaking is hard and complicated. So many factors need to be considered.

I've had the honour of supporting speakers for children's hospitals and patient organizations. Any type of storyteller should be supported. It is best to have a formal structure. This Family Talks program is an example of an initiative supported by paid staff. [115] While having a funded program is ideal, it is not mandatory. Any staff member who has an interest in patient stories can learn to support speakers.

 Make sure someone is assigned to helping the storyteller before, during, and after the session.

This person needs to be willing to do outreach, be a good listener and be aware of their own biases so they can truly coach the storyteller. In sports, the best coaches do not push their own agenda, they encourage the athlete to perform their best.

A public speaking coach can do many things. First, they can act as a liaison between the organizer and the speaker to learn about logistics, key messages, and to gain a good understanding of the audience.

Often health care stories are long and complex. Sometimes people need coaching to go beyond telling a chronological story, to shorten a story and tailor it for an audience. This means sitting with the storyteller and honouring their experience, no matter how long it takes.

 Outreach is crucial to offer safe spaces for folks to tell their intimate stories, sometimes for the first time. Do not ask people to come to a meeting room at the hospital, unless that's where they want to go.

It is only when the entire story is on the table that the work to craft a story for an audience can begin. People can pull out key messages themselves once they have a sense of what the audience's wants and needs are. It is a matter of matching up what the audience needs to hear with what the speaker needs to say. The connecting of the two needs is critical.

As a storyteller, I've been guilty of missing the mark. I haven't acknowledged the audience's concerns before I've launched into my own. I have started out with a negative story, which can shut an audience down to listening. I've said too much when I've felt desperate to impart all my wisdom in a short period of time to an audience I might never speak to again.

I once spent time at a physician's house, looking through her closet with her to help her pick out what to wear for a media event. "What should I wear?" is not a trivial question. Dress like your audience or dress like yourself? Storytellers should wear what they feel comfortable in – business suits are not required. On the other hand, if people are more confident dressing up – go for it.

Talk about public speaking nerves and emotions. It would be unnatural if people weren't nervous before storytelling. As Maria Shriver says, "Anxiety is a glimpse of your own daring."[116]

TED Talks has perpetuated the myth that speakers don't need notes and should memorize their talks. What TED Talks doesn't tell you is that many of their speakers do have notes – you just can't see them because of the way the TED Talk is shot. Notes might be on a teleprompter, or on an iPad off to the side. It was a relief when I read this in TED Talk founder Chris Anderson's book:

"...what matters is that speakers are comfortable and confident, giving the talk in the way that best allows them to focus on what they're passionate about."[117]

The pressure to memorize has led to people putting all their speaking notes on a slide and then reading from the slide. Resources like the *Presentation Zen* book can guide speakers to make more visually appealing and memorable slide decks. [118]

Lean on the power of white space and graphics, not bullets and dense text. Graphic designers can create amazing slide decks for speakers if you have the budget for them.

Logistics matter for storytellers. If they are presenting at your space – a hospital or a conference centre, then treat them as a treasured guest.

Give detailed transit or parking instructions and make
sure to cover those costs. Arrange to meet the storytellers
in a common spot to welcome them. Make sure they feel
settled. Be a friendly face in the audience. Give positive
feedback afterwards.

I've had many fulsome conversations with speakers in parkades
immediately after their talks. For feedback from evaluation forms, I
never cut and paste comments and send them directly to storytellers. They deserve to have constructive feedback shared gently with
them, as they have shared their hearts and wisdom with audiences.

As a speaker, I still learn as I go. Every audience is different and
my evolution as a speaker is not linear. Presenting on-line during
COVID, while wonderfully accessible, also has its challenges.
Often at the end of my talk, I click 'end meeting' and I never hear
back from the organizers. I have no feedback loop, I never know
how my words landed with the audience, who I often can't see on
camera. I can't tell if I've soared or bombed. It teaches me again
how important it is to give storytellers feedback.

 While audiences are given surveys to critique speakers,
don't forget to give the storyteller a chance to share how
the experience was for them. Organizers and coaches
can learn from that feedback too.

Underpinning coaching for storytellers is this: Do people feel
used for their stories? Or are they given the honour and respect
that they deserve?

EVERYBODY HAS A STORY

Once I co-presented to a group of pediatric residents on the family perspective of having a kid in the hospital. I had a number of friendly suggestions about working with families, but after I read the evaluations, I realized I had missed the mark.

"We work really hard. What about us?" said one of the comments. I had not given space to acknowledge the residents' stories.

I did not make that mistake again. I thought about that question for a long time. If I believe in relationship-centred care as I say I do, that means that both parties in the relationship must feel seen and heard.

The audience heard me say: *Me, me, me, this is what I need.* My error was that I did not provide an opportunity for them to tell their own stories.

Begin staff presentations with roundtable introductions and an easy ice-breaker question, like, 'What's your favourite TV show and why?' so that everybody gets a chance to speak. Then pause to ask reflective practice questions where people can either share their stories publicly or keep them just for themselves.

Let us begin with the premise that everybody in health care has a story. Reflective practices like Schwartz Rounds are all about staff storytelling. [119] On Twitter, Dr. Colleen Farrell created #medhumchat, which is, "reflection, empathy, and connection in healthcare through discussions of poetry and prose." [120]

Dr. Rita Charon's Narrative Medicine movement also uses the power of art for clinicians to share their stories.[121] I once heard her speak and wrote about her talk.

"Once we understand how unified we are at the human lived experience, then our troubles (in health care) are over," said Dr. Charon.

She spoke about boundaries, and how the artificial borders we place between each other as 'professionals' and 'patients' are actually permeable. She wondered what methods she could use so she did not have to be a stranger to her patients and concluded that this can only happen when she listens closely to patients with a mixture of curiosity and wonder.

I will repeat the wisdom from Dr. Charon, because this is important: "Pay attention to where the suffering happens. This is where the healing begins."[122]

 Create opportunities for patients and health professionals to share their stories *together*. **Start a book club where everybody is invited to participate.** *Greg's Wings* **is a short film about patient safety that is offered to general audiences.**[123] **There is value in the conversation afterwards in hearing different points of view.**

Co-authoring is a way to tell stories together. In 2017, I wrote an article with radiation therapist Amanda Bolderston about our different perspectives on feedback I had for the cancer hospital.

Amanda explains the concept of narrative inquiry, "...using narratives in health care is not new, there are numerous examples of patient stories, health care professional stories, and health care professional as-patient stories in many formats." What is new are health professionals and patients writing stories together.[124]

Everybody has a story. And everybody has to look after their own hearts so they can look after the hearts of others. This is where compassion is born.

A WELL-TOLD STORY

Here are a few of my tips about storytelling in the professional realm:

1. Keep it real. There is a fine balance between cheerleading and complaining. I share a positive story, then if I have a negative story, I always suggest what could have made it better. Constructive and authentic stories help lift morale and give a sense of hope.

2. In groups, listen more than you talk. Check your own judgment and be as open-hearted as you can when listening to another's story.

3. Be careful of getting stuck in your own story. Sometimes your own story can overshadow or diminish the importance of the stories of the people you serve.

4. A grief counsellor once told me: It is okay for people to have their story, and for you to have your story, and for those two stories to be different.

5. Be wary of comparing or minimizing stories. We don't have to compete with our suffering.

6. Don't steal other people's stories for your own gain – especially people who have less power than you. There are many health professional authors who are guilty of this.

7. Please don't ignore other patient stories if you yourself become a patient. Share the stage and your microphone with others. Nobody's story is more important than someone else's, no matter their title or position.

8. The only person you can represent with your story is your own fine self. Be mindful about speaking on behalf of others. As a mother, I've been guilty of speaking on behalf of my children –

especially my son who has an intellectual disability. I've been working hard to support him to share his own story instead. It is always an honour for me to bear witness to someone's story, no matter who it is. I wish for more safe places where all kinds of people are guided to share their experiences.

In the telling comes the healing. And we all need healing in our own ways.

ART OF STORYTELLING WORKSHOP

Workshops can help people craft their stories. They can be a combination of book readings, videos, a swapping of favourite health care books, podcasts and videos, writing prompts, and small group work. It is great fun to think outside the box with a health care audience who don't yet realize they are all creative beings.

One of my key messages about crafting stories is to 'know thy audience.' Each of my workshops are tailored for different audiences for that very reason.

Folks who work in health care share patient stories for teaching or clinical reasons, but I'm interested in supporting health care staff to understand their *own* personal stories about their passion for health care. These are a type of origin story. Reconnecting with why they chose health care is a powerful thing and essential for any reflective practice.

Why tell stories of any kind – whether they are written, the spoken word, or in visual form? Well, as I say, if you touch hearts, you can change minds.

I believe stories go beyond sharing an experience. An experience tends to be chronological (this happened, then this, then this). A story includes experience for context, but the crucial part of the story is the reflective piece. This happened, here is why it mattered to me and here is what I want you, as the audience or reader, to take away. (My brilliant book editor, Mish Phillips, taught me this).

The human aspect of stories show that we all have more in common with each other than we have differences. Crafting a story with impact has common elements. Here are the basics of storytelling in five points:

1. Understand your intention or your 'why.'
2. Know thy audience.
3. Craft three key messages.
4. Hone your approach.
5. Identify what you want your audience to take away.

Stories do not have to be limited to the written word or told behind a podium. Art is a clever way to tell a story – through photography, film, visual art, music, or poetry. Art can heal in any form it takes.

The topics for storytelling workshops are endless. You can chat about the nuts and bolts of writing a story (English 101); share public speaking tips; explain how to use humour in storytelling; talk about coaching storytellers and crafting hard stories for constructive feedback, advocacy, and teaching purposes.

You can discuss the ethics of stories, including 'how does your story change over time' and 'whose story is it?' There is writing stories just for yourself and writing to get published or to speak in public – and how to find those opportunities.

You can explore how you are honouring the storytellers and examine the responsibility audiences have when they listen to stories. Then there is the art behind coaching folks to work with the media (top hint: don't wear stripes on camera).

Anne Lamott does the best job of explaining storytelling: "Shitty first drafts. Butt in chair. Just do it. You own everything that happened to you."[125]

The most important thing is simply to start. Don't wait for the perfect time, for there is no such thing as a perfect time.

WHAT ELSE HEALS

My thing is the written word, so I talk a lot about storytelling. Think of what creative pursuits light you up and how it intersects with health care. That's the place to start.

I dabbled in poetry when I stumbled upon a poetry class at our local arts centre. I liked the stripped-down nature of this genre, which helped me get to the point more quickly than my long, rambling journal entries. If you don't consider yourself a writer, perhaps you are a poet instead?

If words aren't your jam, with cameras on our phones, photography is an easily accessible way to tell our stories. There are many examples of disability and health stories told through photography on Instagram, including Katie Jameson, who documents her life as a mother of a young girl with Down syndrome. Danielle Doby is a high-profile author who has breast cancer and documents her patient experiences through photographs too.[126, 127]

If organizations truly want to hear a variety of stories from diverse people, they must break free from the podium. If they want diversity in speakers, they need to create safe spaces for different kinds of stories. The experiences that are shared holding a microphone while talking to slides are only one way to tell a story.

It is not a coincidence that leaning on the humanities helps nurture humanity in health care. Academically, humanity includes areas like fine art, literature, drama, music, gender studies, and philosophy. Why are health faculties – which reside in the sciences – traditionally divorced from the humanities, except for an obligatory English class for students?

If you want change, you must do something different than what has been done before. If health care is both an art and a science, then students should be exposed to both.

We need to look to the arts in clinical practice in order to be more human for both patients and staff. There are a handful of health specialties that do the fine work of focusing on the arts: therapists in music, art and recreation, pet therapy, therapeutic clowns. Some hospitals feature art galleries. Alas, these positions and initiatives are rare and often precarious because they are funded by foundation or grants. Acknowledging the importance of the arts in health care means they have a line in the operational budget.

It is relatively easy to embed the arts into health care – if there's a will, there's a way. Hush Foundation was started by Dr. Catherine Crock in Melbourne, Australia. She recognized that stress levels were high at the children's hospital where she did bone marrow procedures and lumbar punctures on young patients with cancer.

Dr. Crock led Hush's initiative for classical and jazz music composers to create and record soothing music for waiting rooms and operating theatres.

> *"Working alongside anaesthetists in the development of new pain relief systems for these young patients, Dr. Crock sought to reduce the stress and anxiety felt by patients, families and staff...through the use of especially composed music from some of Australia's foremost musicians and composers. The music helps evoke a sense of calm and optimism."[128]*

Music is part of an environment and can be calming for both staff and patients. The Hush Foundation believes in transforming the culture of health care through the arts.

For the past twenty years, Dr. Crock – yes, the same doctor whose couch I sat on in Melbourne at the beginning of this book – has championed the use of calming music to reduce stress and anxiety. She has led the creation of 19 volumes of music that are composed for health care environments.[129]

Music today is accessible – you do not need a CD player to listen to music. A phone with an account to a streaming service, hooked up to headphones or a speaker system works.

A few years ago, I got my hand on a Hush CD and offered it to the manager of a clinic. They had a waiting area for families that was stark and silent. I was hoping they would try out the music, just to see the response. The CD sat on a shelf, never used. The reason given was that, 'some children are agitated by music,' and 'not everybody likes classical music,' So there was no music at all.

 If you have a waiting area, walk into it during a busy time. Listen. These areas are never silent. Be a secret shopper and check it out. Often the sounds are the receptionist talking to patients on the phone. Try playing calming music and see what happens.

The arts can offer other gifts to health care: books, poetry, plays, films, videos, and visual arts.

Hush Foundation has added health care plays to its portfolio of ways to lean on the humanities in health care. Their plays are about patient safety and the culture of bullying in health care. Plays are stories that have come to life and can be a powerful mechanism to help staff feel compassion for patients, other staff, and themselves.[130]

We will all need health care at some point in our lives. After medical treatment, we will need support to heal. Now is the time to think seriously and creatively about healing.

Visual artist Ted Meyer has a TED talk called *A Portrait of a*

Patient Experience, where he describes his art projects, which involve painting scars. "People always say – art should be about something until art is about something and then they don't really want to look at it," he says.[131]

Is that the reason for the reluctance to embrace the arts in health care, because art about illness is too painful to look at?

There are champions in this area. Some hospitals employ artists-in-residence, and many other health care facilities dedicate space for art galleries – or at least have original art on their walls. Artists or musicians in residence can provide therapy for inpatients and consult about integrating art into clinical environments.[132]

Think beyond the podium to consider what a story looks like. It might be poetry, photography, visual art, music, or film. Embracing a variety of ways to share patient experience will help you also embrace all kinds of patients.

When I need a respite from this difficult world, I lean on the arts and humanities. The mashing up of art with health care ultimately makes health care more human.

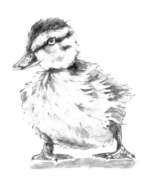

PART 4

CONCLUSION:
MY SCHITT'S CREEK

W hat does health care reimagined look like? Funnily enough, my ideal world is depicted in a TV show that isn't about health care at all.

Schitt's Creek is a Canadian sitcom that aired from 2015 to 2020 which became widely popular beyond Canada's borders. It is about a wealthy family who loses their money and, destitute, has to move to a small town. This change in circumstances forces them to consider what is important in life, and the family learns the real meaning of humility, love, and community.

The documentary *Best Wishes, Warmest Regards: A Schitt's Creek Farewell* explains its success. What Dan and Eugene Levy did with *Schitt's Creek* was to show the world they wanted to see: one of caring and compassion. The series depicted a realistic utopia of how life could be if we were open-hearted.[133]

> *"Schitt's Creek presents a better world than we*
> *live in. We aren't teaching them a lesson. We are*
> *showing them what life could look like." - Dan Levy*

Schitt's Creek is the world of health care that I'd like to see.

We need to reimagine health care to build the health care system we want to see. This book has dug into the problems, the what is wrong: the power imbalances, the insistence on efficiency, the lack of focus on care. But I also offered solutions based on my work experience and my bird's eye view wisdom from being a patient and caregiver in the health system.

Everybody says that health care is complex. It doesn't need to be that way. If the root of health care is caring for each other, then all policies, operational processes and individual decisions – need to be guided by that philosophy.

My *Schitt's Creek* for health care is that all people are seen as human beings first, not roles or diagnoses. Creativity and the arts are embraced. Administrators take off their business suits and go to the people. Feedback is welcomed and acted upon.

Revisiting the title of this book, will health care ever get its ducks in a row? Dr. Rod Phillips, my insightful friend who helped me in the introduction, suggested this will not happen until patients are meaningfully included in decisions that affect them. I agree that partnering with patients should not be an afterthought, as it is now. It needs to be the foundation of all policy and process decisions.

However, humans are not rubber ducks, all identical and ready to be lined up. Considering that human beings are distinct creatures, maybe a perfect arrangement of ducks is not the metaphor we need. With diverse mama ducks as our symbolic leaders, we can reimagine health care together in our own unique, dishevelled, and human ways.

Look at the ducks on this book's cover. One duck looks mad. Another one is squawking to herself. One is marching forward confidently while another is heading sideways and has seemingly lost their way. The little duck at the top is just starting out and waiting patiently for guidance.

Health care is about caring for humans. There is a messiness that goes along with that. Ducklings are chaotic, as are people. They have minds of their own and distinct personalities.

Your ducks cannot and will not be neatly lined up.

We all have the ability to be leaders, irrespective of our credentials or fancy titles. As individuals, we have the power to do something, without waiting for the system to change.

Go to the people. Allow safe spaces for stories and feedback. Use the magic of the arts to soften health care. Embrace this messiness, for humans are squawky, wonderful, and imperfect creatures.

Let us follow each other towards the light and forge a new path – where health care is firmly rooted in love.

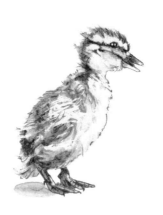

NOTES

INTRODUCTION

1. *The Many Faces of Patient Engagement*. Gallivan, Kovacs Burns, Bellows and Eigenseher. 2012. participatorymedicine.org/journal/evidence/research/2012/12/26/the-many-faces-of-patient-engagement/

2. *Patients Included*. patientsincluded.org

3. *Relationship-centred care: Toward real health system reform*. Van Aerde. 2015. cjpl.ca/relationship.html

4. *What it means to "hold space" for people, plus eight tips on how to do it well*. Heather Plett. 2015. heatherplett.com/2015/03/hold-space/

POWER TO THE PEOPLE

HEALTH CARE IS NOT A CAR FACTORY

5. *The Checklist Manifesto*. Atul Gawande. 2009. atulgawande.com/book/the-checklist-manifesto/

6. *Lean management in health care: definition, concepts, methodology and effects reported*. Adegboyega et al. ncbi.nlm.nih.gov/pmc/articles/PMC4171573/

7. *PTSD in the hospital: Why the emotional scars of serious illnesses linger long after treatment*. *White Coat, Black Art podcast*. 2018. cbc.ca/radio/whitecoat/ptsd-in-the-hospital-why-the-emotional-scars-of-serious-illnesses-linger-long-after-treatment-1.4590370

8. *Lean Six Sigma Green Belt for Healthcare*. McGill University. mcgill.ca/desautels/gmscm/program-operations-excellence/lean-six-sigma-healthcare

9. *Why We Revolt*. Victor Montori. 2017. patientrevolution.org/whywerevolt

THE UGLY UNDERBELLY

10. *Neglected No More: The Urgent Need to Improve the Lives of Canada's Elders in the Wake of a Pandemic*. André Picard. 2021. penguinrandomhouse.ca/books/669793/neglected-no-more-by-andre-picard/9780735282247

11. *All of our tanks are on empty*. The Gritty Nurse Podcast. 2021. grittynurse.com/podcast/episode/b078a32f/all-of-our-tanks-are-on-empty-discussing-tangible-mental-health-tools-for-healthcare-providers-with-dr-jason-harley

12. *Death of Mrs. Joyce Echaquan, coroner's investigation report*. 2021. coroner.gouv.qc.ca/medias/communiques/detail-dun-communique/466.html

13. *80-year-old kicked out of hospital for holding husband's hand*. CBC News. 2021. cbc.ca/news/canada/new-brunswick/kim-crevatin-moncton-hospital-visitors-covid-alzheimers-1.5915184

DANCING WITH THE SHIRTLESS GUY

14. *First Follower: Leadership Lessons from Dancing Guy*. 2010. youtube.com/watch?v=fW8amMCVAJQ

LET US GET TO MAYBE

15. *A Litany for Survival*. Audre Lorde. 1978. poetryfoundation.org/poems/147275/a-litany-for-survival

16. *Getting to Maybe: How the World is Changed.* Frances Westley, Brenda Zimmerman & Michael Patton. 2007. penguinrandomhouse.ca/books/189202/getting-to-maybe-by-frances-westley-brenda-zimmerman-and-michael-patton/9780679314448

17. *Toyota Production System.* global.toyota/en/company/vision-and-philosophy/production-system/

18. *Turning to One Another: Simple Conversations to Restore Hope to the Future.* Margaret J. Wheatley. 2009. margaretwheatley.com/books-products/books/

19. *Embers: One Ojibway's Meditations.* Richard Wagamese. 2016. douglas-mcintyre.com/products/9781771621335

20. David Whyte. davidwhyte.com

21. *Love, no matter what.* Andrew Solomon. 2013. ted.com/talks/andrew_solomon_love_no_matter_what?language=en

22. *How great leaders inspire action.* Simon Sinek. 2009. ted.com/talks/simon_sinek_how_great_leaders_inspire_action?language=en

23. *The power of vulnerability.* Brené Brown. 2010. ted.com/talks/brene_brown_the_power_of_vulnerability?language=en

24. *Empathy: The Human Connection to Patient Care.* 2013. youtube.com/watch?v=cDDWvj_q-o8

ROOTED IN LOVE

25. *Gathering of Kindness.* gatheringofkindness.org

26. *Bird's Eye View: Stories of a life lived in health care.* Sue Robins. 2019. suerobins.com/books

RELATIONSHIP CENTRED CARE

27. *Relationship-centred care: Toward real health system reform.* Van Aerde. 2015. cjpl.ca/relationship.html

DON'T GIVE THEM ALL OF YOUR HEART

28. Institute for Patient- and Family-Centered Care. ipfcc.org

HUMANITY IN HEALTH CARE FOR ALL

29. *Love: A word that medicine fears.* Kirsten Meisinger. 2012. kevinmd.com/blog/2012/11/love-word-medicine-fears.html

HUMANS, NOT HEROES

30. *We Are All Perfectly Fine: A Memoir of Love, Medicine and Healing.* Jillian Horton. 2021. harpercollins. ca/9781443461641/we-are-all-perfectly-fine/

DO YOU VALUE ALL PATIENTS?

31. *Diversity of U.S. Medical Students by Parental Income.* Jolly. 2008. aamc.org/media/5776/download

32. *An uneven recovery: Measuring COVID-19 vaccine equity in Ontario.* Iveniuk, Leon. 2021. wellesleyinstitute.com/ wp-content/uploads/2021/04/An-uneven-recovery-Mea-suring-COVID-19-vaccine-equity-in-Ontario.pdf

33. *Global COVID-19 vaccine inequity.* Burki. 2021. thelancet.com/ journals/laninf/article/PIIS1473-3099(21)00344-3/fulltext

34. *Including People with Developmental Disabilities as a Priority Group in Canada's COVID-19 Vaccination Program: Key Considerations.* Campanella et al. 2021. porticonetwork. ca/web/hcardd/news/-/blogs/research-evidence-regard-ing-covid-19-and-developmental-disabilities

JOY AT WORK

35. *Sickboy* podcast. sickboypodcast.com

36. *The Boy in the Moon*. Ian Brown. 2010. penguinrandomhouse.ca/books/19492/the-boy-in-the-moon-by-ianbrown/9780679310099

37. *The Spirit Catches You and You Fall Down: A Hmong Child, Her American Doctors, and the Collision of Two Cultures*. Anne Fadiman. 1997. us.macmillan.com/books/9780374533403/the-spirit-catches-you-and-you-fall-down

REFLECTIONS ON REFLECTIVE PRACTICE

38. *Gibb's Reflective Cycle*. Reflection Toolkit, the University of Edinburgh. ed.ac.uk/reflection/reflectors-toolkit/reflecting-on-experience/gibbs-reflective-cycle

39. *Schwartz Rounds and Membership*. The Schwarz Center. theschwartzcenter.org/programs/schwartz-rounds/

40. *Code Lavender: A tool for staff support*. Stone. 2018. my.clevelandclinic.org/-/scassets/files/org/locations/hillcrest-hospital/spiritual-services/code-lavender.ashx

WE ALL HAVE STORIES

41. Gathering of Kindness. gatheringofkindness.org

42. *Narrative Medicine: A Model for Empathy, Reflection, Profession, and Trust*. Charon. 2001. jamanetwork.com/journals/jama/fullarticle/194300

43. *Pay attention to where the suffering happens*. Sue Robins. 2016. suerobins.wordpress.com/2016/04/10/pay-attention-to-where-the-suffering-happens

HEALTH CARE REIMAGINED

44. *The Serenity Prayer and Me*. alcoholics-anonymous.org.uk/
    Members/Fellowship-Magazines/SHARE-Magazine/De-
    cember-2019/The-Serenity-Prayer-and-Me

45. *Matters of Life and Death*. André Picard. 2017. andrepicard.
    com/books

46. *Why We Revolt*. Victor Montori. 2017. patientrevolution.
    org/whywerevolt

START HERE FOR MEANINGFUL ENGAGEMENT

47. Patients Included. patientsincluded.org

48. Planetree International. planetree.org

49. The Beryl Institute. theberylinstitute.org

50. Institute for Patient- and Family-Centered Care. ipfcc.org

51. Gathering of Kindness. gatheringofkindness.org

52. The Patient Experience Library. patientlibrary.net

53. *Inadmissible Evidence*. The Patient Experience Li-
    brary. 2020. patientlibrary.net/cgi-bin/library.
    cgi?page=Blog;top=184

KITCHEN TABLE REVOLUTION

54. *Promising Care*. Donald M. Berwick. 2013. wiley.com/
    en-us/Promising+Care%3A+How+We+Can+Res-
    cue+Health+Care+by+Improving+It-p-9781118795880

THE D WORD

55. *Understanding and Using Health Experiences: Improv-
    ing patient care*. Sue Ziebland, Angela Coulter, Joseph
    D. Calabrese & Louise Locock. 2013. oxford.univer-
    sitypressscholarship.com/view/10.1093/acprof:o-

so/9780199665372.001.0001/acprof-9780199665372

56. Amy Ma. @Ctzen_Improver. https://twitter.com/Ctzen_ Improver

57. *The Racist Lady with the Lamp*. Natalie Stake-Doucet. 2020. historynewsnetwork.org/article/178101

58. *William Osler: saint in a "White man's dominion"*. Nav Persaud, Heather Butts and Philip Berger. 2020. cmaj.ca/content/192/45/E1414

59. *What patients wish health professionals knew about partnering with them*. Diana Duong. 2021. cmaj.ca/content/193/27/E1056

60. *A cluster randomized controlled trial to increase breast cancer screening among African American women: the black cosmetologists promoting health program*. Sadler et al. 2011. europepmc.org/article/pmc/pmc4153602

61. Conference proceedings from the Montreal Children's Hospital 30th anniversary of the Socio-cultural and Interpreter Services – 2018 initiative.

TWO STEPS BACKWARDS

62. *KGH introduces flexible visiting hours*. Kingston General Hospital. 2009. cfhi-fcass.ca/sf-docs/default-source/patient-engagement/info-memo.pdf

63. *80-year-old kicked out of hospital for holding husband's hand*. CBC News. 2021. cbc.ca/news/canada/new-brunswick/ kim-crevatin-moncton-hospital-visitors-covid-alzheimers-1.5915184

64. *Woman with disability dies alone at B.C. hospital amid COVID-19 restrictions*. CBC News. 2020. cbc.ca/news/canada/british-columbia/woman-disability-dies-white-rock-hospital-covid-19-1.5543468

65. *Safely Re-entering Long-Term Care Homes During COVID-19: A Resource for Essential Care Partners. Healthcare Excellence Canada.* 2020. healthcareexcellence.ca/en/what-we-do/what-we-do-together/safely-re-entering-long-term-care-homes-during-covid-19/

THE ART OF REALLY LISTENING

66. *Bird's Eye View: Stories of a life lived in health care.* Sue Robins. 2019. suerobins.com/books

67. *Krebs Cycle.* ScienceDirect. sciencedirect.com/topics/engineering/krebs-cycle

68. *There's no such thing as the perfect child.* Sue Robins. 2010. theglobeandmail.com/life/facts-and-arguments/theres-no-such-thing-as-the-perfect-child/article1214545/

69. *The CARE Method of Screening ACEs: How and Why to Ask Adult Patients about Childhood Adversity.* 2019. youtube.com/watch?v=fc7NBdCYUAE

70. *Compassionomics: The Revolutionary Scientific Evidence that Caring Makes a Difference.* Stephen Trzeciak. 2019. compassionomics.com

WORK IS WORK IS WORK

71. *Patient partner compensation in research and health care: the patient perspective on why and how.* Richards et al. 2018. pxjournal.org/cgi/viewcontent.cgi?article=1334&context=journal

WAITING ROOM EXPERIENCE

72. *Bird's Eye View: Stories of a life lived in health care.* Sue Robins. 2019. suerobins.com/books

LOW HANGING FRUIT

73. *Putting Patients First: Best Practices in Patient-Centered Care, 2nd edition.* Editors Susan B. Frampton, Patrick A. Charmel. 2008. wiley.com/en-ca/Putting+Patients+-First%3A+Best+Practices+in+Patient+Centered+-Care%2C+2nd+Edition-p-9780470377024

74. *Do bedside whiteboards enhance communication in hospitals? An exploratory multimethod study of patient and nurse perspectives.* Goyal et al. 2019. pubmed.ncbi.nlm.nih.gov/31694874/

STAY CURIOUS RESEARCHERS

75. *Patient Engagement in Health Research: A How-to Guide for Researchers.* Alberta SPOR Support Unit. 2018. albertainnovates.ca/wp-content/uploads/2018/06/How-To-Guide-Researcher-Version-8.0-May-2018.pdf

76. *How can we make the partnership with patients and families more impactful?* Canadian Patient Safety Institute. 2015. patientsafetyinstitute.ca/en/toolsResources/Pages/How-can-we-make-the-partnership-with-patients-families-more-impactful.aspx

77. *It Doesn't Have to Hurt. A patient-oriented research program in children's pain management.* itdoesnthavetohurt.ca

78. *Journal of Family Nursing.* journals.sagepub.com/home/jfn

79. *Journal of Medical Imaging and Radiation Sciences.* jmirs.org/content/authorinfo

WHAT IS COUNTED, COUNTS

80. *Bird's Eye View: Stories of a life lived in health care.* Sue Robins. 2019. suerobins.com/books

81. *The Patient Experience Library.* patientlibrary.net/cgi-bin/documents.cgi

82. *Sharing patient stories openly.* James Munro. 2020. careopinion.org.uk/blogposts/850/sharing-patient-stories-openly

83. Care Opinion. careopinion.org.uk/info/about

84. *Using Care Opinion in teaching - simple ideas for getting started.* James Munro. 2020. careopinion.org.uk/resources/site?id=blog-resources/1-files/using-care-opinion-in-teaching---simple-ideas-for-getting-started.pdf

85. *A safe space: Indigenous doctor creates online platform to empower racialized patients in health system.* Canadian Medical Association staff. 2021. boldly.cma.ca/blog/indigenous-doctor-creates-online-platform-to-empower-racialized-patients-in-health-system

86. *Promising Care.* Donald M. Berwick. 2013. wiley.com/en-us/Promising+Care%3A+How+We+Can+Rescue+Health+Care+by+Improving+It-p-9781118795880

87. *Researcher develops patient-reported compassion measure for health care.* Brennan Black. N.d. nursing.ucalgary.ca/news/researcher-develops-patient-reported-compassion-measure-health-care

88. *Measuring compassionate healthcare with the 12-item Schwartz Center Compassionate Care Scale.* Rodriguez and Lown. 2019. pubmed.ncbi.nlm.nih.gov/31487300/

89. Picker. picker.org/working-with-us/surveys/

YOU CAN'T HANDLE THE TRUTH

90. *Death of Mrs. Joyce Echaquan, coroner's investigation report.* 2021. coroner.gouv.qc.ca/medias/communiques/detail-dun-communique/466.html

91. *A Legacy of Mistrust: Can Indigenous Health Care in BC's North Turn a Corner?* The Tyee. 2021. thetyee.ca/News/2021/05/17/Legacy-Mistrust-Indigenous-Health-Care-BC-North/?utm_source=weekly&utm_medium=email&utm_campaign=170521

92. *Betrayal Trauma.* Erin Gilmer. 2020. healthasahumanright.wordpress.com/2020/12/07/betrayal-trauma/#more-2539

93. *Caring for care: Online feedback in the context of public healthcare services.* Mazanderani et al. 2021. sciencedirect.com/science/article/abs/pii/S0277953621006122?dgcid=author

94. *The Wounded Storyteller: Body, Illness, and Ethics, 2nd edition.* Arthur W. Frank. 2013. press.uchicago.edu/ucp/books/book/chicago/W/bo14674212.html

95. Alan Alda Center for Communicating Science. aldacenter.org/about/our_history.php

96. *Science, in the Words of Alan Alda.* The Atlantic. 2015. theatlantic.com/education/archive/2015/01/science-in-the-words-of-alan-alda/384218/

THE GOOD, THE BAD AND THE UGLY

97. *Difficult families?* Marianne Selby-Boothroyd and Liz Wilson. N.d. certitude.london/difficult-families/

98. *How We Go From Competent Caregiver to 'Family From Hell'.* Donna Thomson. 2017. donnathomson.com/2017/11/how-we-go-from-competent-caregiver-to.html?spref=tw

NURTURE THE HUMANITIES

99. *The introduction of medical humanities in the undergraduate curriculum of Greek medical schools: challenge and necessity.* Batistatou et al. 2010. ncbi.nlm.nih.gov/pmc/articles/PMC3031316/

TELLING OUR UNTOLD STORIES

100. *Promising Care*. Donald M. Berwick. 2013. wiley.com/en-us/Promising+Care%3A+How+We+Can+Rescue+Health+Care+by+Improving+It-p-9781118795880

101. *Inadmissible Evidence*. The Patient Experience Library. 2020. patientlibrary.net/cgi-bin/library.cgi?page=Blog;top=184

102. *The Big Sick*. 2017. imdb.com/title/tt5462602

103. *Sickboy* podcast. sickboypodcast.com/

104. *Happy Faces Only: The Story of a Little Girl who Lived*. Karen Klak. 2021. karenklak.com/happy-faces-only

105. *"Good" and "bad" are incomplete stories we tell ourselves*. Heather Lanier. 2017. ted.com/talks/heather_lanier_good_and_bad_are_incomplete_stories_we_tell_ourselves#t-3343

106. *Your Silence Will Not Protect You*. Audre Lorde. 2017. silverpress.org/collections/all-products

DO NO HARM

107. *Three Sides to Every Story: Preparing Patient and Family Storytellers, Facilitators, and Audiences*. Hawthornthwaite et al. 2018. thepermanentejournal.org/issues/64-the-permanente-journal/narrative-medicine/6693-three-sides-to-every-story-preparing-patient-and-family-storytellers,-facilitators,-and-audiences.html

STORIES AS HEALING

108. *Bird's Eye View: Stories of a life lived in health care*. Sue Robins. 2019. suerobins.com/books

109. *The power of storytelling*. The Health Foundation. 2016. health.org.uk/newsletter-feature/power-of-storytelling

110. *Patients' stories in healthcare curricula: learning the art*

of healthcare practice with patients. Yan Wong, Job & Anstey. 2018. tandfonline.com/doi/full/10.1080/030987 7X.2019.1596234

111. *Storytelling as a research tool and intervention around public health perceptions and behaviour: a protocol for a systematic narrative review.* McCall et al. 2019 bmjopen.bmj.com/content/9/12/e030597

112. *Determining Patient Readiness to Share Their Healthcare Stories: A Tool for Prospective Patient Storytellers to Determine Their Readiness to Discuss Their Healthcare Experiences.* Ashdown and Maniate. 2020. researchgate.net/publication/343928193_Determining_Patient_Readiness_to_Share_Their_Healthcare_Stories_A_Tool_for_Prospective_Patient_Storytellers_to_Determine_Their_Readiness_to_Discuss_Their_Healthcare_Experiences

113. *Beyond catharsis: the nuanced emotion of patient storytellers in an educational role.* Roebotham et al. 2018. researchgate.net/publication/323127597_Beyond_catharsis_the_nuanced_emotion_of_patient_storytellers_in_an_educational_role

114. *The Wounded Storyteller: Body, Illness, and Ethics, 2nd edition.* Arthur W. Frank. 2013. press.uchicago.edu/ucp/books/book/chicago/W/bo14674212.html

COACHING STORYTELLERS

115. *Stollery Children's Hospital's Family Talks program.* Hospital News. N.d. hospitalnews.com/stollery-childrens-hosptials-family-talks-program/

116. *And One More Thing Before You Go...* Maria Shriver. 2007. simonandschuster.com/books/And-One-More-Thing-Before-You-Go/Maria-Shriver/9780743281034

117. *TED Talks: The Official TED Guide to Public Speaking.* Chris

Anderson. 2016. ted.com/read/ted-talks-the-official-ted-guide-to-public-speaking

118. Presentation Zen. presentationzen.com

EVERYBODY HAS A STORY

119. *Schwartz Rounds and Membership.* The Schwarz Center. theschwartzcenter.org/programs/schwartz-rounds

120. *Medical Humanities Chat.* @MedHumChat. twitter.com/medhumchat

121. *Narrative Medicine*, Columbia University. sps.columbia.edu/academics/masters/narrative-medicine

122. *Pay attention to where the suffering happens.* Sue Robins. 2016. suerobins.wordpress.com/2016/04/10/pay-attention-to-where-the-suffering-happens

123. Greg's Wings. gregswings.ca

124. *The Radiation Therapist and the Patient: Epiphanies, Stories, and Social Media.* Bolderston and Robins. 2018. jmirs.org/article/S1939-8654(17)30292-8/pdf

ART OF STORYTELLING WORKSHOP

125. *Anne Lamott shares all that she knows: "Everyone is screwed up, broken, clingy, and scared".* Anne Lamott. 2015. salon.com/2015/04/10/anne_lamott_shares_all_that_she_knows_everyone_is_screwed_up_broken_clingy_and_scared

WHAT ELSE HEALS

126. Katie Jameson. katie_jameson. instagram.com/katie__jameson

127. Danielle Doby. daniellledoby. instagram.com/danielledoby

128. *The health care pioneer. Engaging Women.* N.d. engaging-

women.com.au/stories/dr-catherine-crock

129. The Hush Foundation. hush.org.au

130. *Our Healthcare Plays*. The Hush Foundation. hush.org.au/our-healthcare-plays

131. *A portrait of the patient experience*. 2017. youtube.com/watch?v=g_HOIg1qV9A

132. Smith Center for Healing and the Arts. smithcenter.org/arts-healing/artist-in-residence-program

CONCLUSION: MY SCHITT'S CREEK

133. *Best Wishes, Warmest Regards: A Schitt's Creek Farewell*. 2020. imdb.com/title/tt12004838/?ref_=fn_al_tt_1

BONUS NOTES

These resources about Equity, Diversity and Inclusion (EDI) have been generously shared by Amy Ma, to supplement her interview from *The D Word* chapter.

The Principles of Trustworthiness. Center For Health Justice, Association of American Medical Colleges. aamchealthjustice.org/resources/trustworthiness-toolkit

Complaint as Diversity Work. 2018. youtube.com/watch?v=JQ_1k-FwkfVE

Beyond Cultural Safety in Palliative Care: How to be an Anti-Racist Palliative Care Clinician. Amy Tan and Alexandra Dobie. 2021. speakingofmedicine.plos.org/2021/08/03/beyond-cultural-safety-in-palliative-care-how-to-be-an-anti-racist-palliative-care-clinician/

Critical race theory in medicine. CMAJ Podcasts (Canadian

Medical Association Journal). 2021. soundcloud.com/cmajpod-casts/210178-medsoc

Unique premed program teaches new approach to race and health. Jim Patterson. 2017. news.vanderbilt.edu/2017/09/20/unique-premed-race-health/

The Pathophysiology of Racial Disparities. Amanda Calhoun. 2021. nejm.org/doi/full/10.1056/NEJMpv2105339

The intersection of race and disability. Indianapolis Recorder. 2021. indianapolisrecorder.com/the-intersection-of-race-and-disability/

If There's Only One Woman in Your Candidate Pool, There's Statistically No Chance She'll Be Hired. Stefanie K. Johnson, David R. Hekman, and Elsa T. Chan. 2016. hbr.org/2016/04/if-theres-on-ly-one-woman-in-your-candidate-pool-theres-statistically-no-chance-shell-be-hired

The Role of Psychological Safety in Diversity and Inclusion. Amy C. Edmondston. 2020. psychologytoday.com/intl/blog/the-fear-less-organization/202006/the-role-psychological-safety-in-diver-sity-and-inclusion

We Don't Need More "Invitations to the Table." We Need a New Ta-ble. Charles Marohn. 2020. strongtowns.org/journal/2020/6/22/invitations-to-the-table

Restructure Your Organization to Actually Advance Racial Justice. Evelyn R. Carter. 2020. hbr.org/2020/06/restructure-your-organi-zation-to-actually-advance-racial-justice

Matters of Engagement podcast, various episodes, https://mattersofengagement.com/democratic-patient-led-councils-the-rise-of-patient-engagement-and-the-erosion-of-advocacy-with-lucy-costa/ and https://mattersofengagement.com/dilem-mas-of-representation-with-paula-rowland/

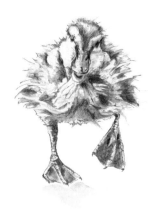

ACKNOWLEDGEMENTS

This book was written to honour my dear friend Mary Morgan, who left this Earth in April 2021. Mary taught me to stand up for what I believe in, but not to forget to live a life of joy.

I want to thank the people who have influenced my thinking over the years about what matters in health care.

The original Stollery Children's Hospital gang championed family-centred care and featured this group of fierce bears: Sharon Willey, Tiffany Keiller, Karen Calhoun, Karen Klak, Cathy Laycock, Angie Christman, Marni Panas, Christina Herbers and Katharina Staub.

Laurene Black, Heather Mattson McCrady, Dawn Wrightson, Jennifer Gallivan and Kathy Reid were staff pioneers who dared to dance on the hill to nurture safe spaces for family and youth voices in their hospital.

I'm forever grateful to Dr. Catherine Crock for role modelling what kindness looks like in real life. She also introduced me to her husband, Dr. Rod Phillips, who inspired the title of this book. Amy Maddison and Kathryn Anderson are part of Cath's Gathering of Kindness team, and I appreciate their gentle and enthusiastic support of my work.

I learned much about staff engagement from hospital managers Lesley Howie, Rita Janke, Tracy Conway, Alda Antunes Silvestre and Kim Tully. Karen Hodge, Jill Howey, and Andrea Ryce took me under their wings at their hospital when I moved provinces to continue my family engagement work.

I'd like to especially recognize colleague and friend Amy Ma for her generous contributions to *The D Word* chapter in this book.

For the folks who made the time to read *Ducks in a Row* and write an endorsement – all champions in their own right – I thank you. A deep bow to all the people I referenced in this book, as their work has greatly contributed to increasing humanity in health care.

I am grateful to my production team: My publisher and agent extraordinaire Mike Waddingham at Bird Communications; and Michelle Phillips, Lexi Wright and Ben Phillips at Hambone Publishing. The look and finesse in this book is due to the talents of illustrator Jacqueline Robins; graphic designer Bobbie Mumby; editor Tara Hogue Harris; researcher Aaron Loehrlein and photographer Ryan Walter Wagner.

My family owns a big piece of my heart. To my adult children Isaac, Ella, and Aaron, your mama loves you very much. Keep going forth and being you. To my brand new grandbaby Levi, keep on shining your light and joy on the world.

To my husband/partner/love of my life Mike, you are the one who helped me bloom. You gave me the soft landing and unconditional love that I've been searching for my whole life. Xo.

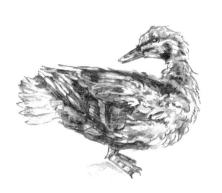

ABOUT THE AUTHOR

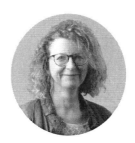

Sue Robins is a health care activist, patient experience champion and a Fellow with Victor Montori's Patient Revolution.

She is a storytelling coach, workshop facilitator, seasoned speaker and health care communications consultant. Her first book *Bird's Eye View: Stories of a life lived in health care* was launched at the Gathering of Kindness in Australia in November 2019.

Her writing has been published in the New York Times, Huffington Post, The Globe and Mail and the Canadian Medical Association Journal.

Sue has experience in paid positions in family engagement at two pediatric hospitals in Canada.

In her health care activism work, Sue co-pilots the Ready For My Shot campaign, an initiative aimed at encouraging people with developmental disabilities to get their COVID vaccine.

Sue is the proud mom of Isaac, Ella and Aaron. She co-owns Bird Communications with her husband Mike. She lives on the ancestral and unceded homelands of the Coast Salish people from the Musqueam, Squamish, and Tsleil-Waututh First Nations.

CONNECT WITH SUE

Join me on social media!

🐦 : twitter.com/suerobinsyvr

📷 : instagram.com/suerobinsbooks

in : linkedin.com/in/sue-robins-6609147

To learn more about Sue's speaking and workshop offerings, please visit **SueRobins.com**

MORE GREAT READS FROM SUE ROBINS

FOR STORY LOVERS:

bird's eye view

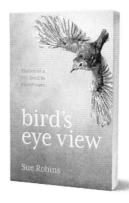

Stories of a life lived in health care.

Bird's Eye View is a compelling book of stories sharing a life lived in health care. Poignant and provocative, Sue's first book highlights the patient and family experience, and includes practical wisdom to inspire us all.

Bird's Eye View can be found on Amazon, Google Books, Apple iBooks, Kobo, Nook and in other leading retail and academic bookstores.

Details on all of Sue's books, including upcoming releases and promotions, can be found at SueRobins.com/books.

MORE GREAT READS FROM SUE ROBINS

FOR HEALTH EDUCATORS:

little bird

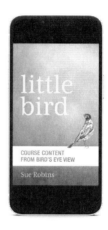

An eBook of Course Content
based on Bird's Eye View

Little Bird is packed with lesson plans and special content that make it a must read for health educators, students and clinicians.

This free eBook is specially designed to be read on an iPhone or Android device, making it a practical reference that can be accessed anywhere.

Little Bird can be found on Amazon, Google Books, Apple, iBooks, Kobo, and Nook – or downloaded directly from SueRobins.com/books.

Manufactured by Amazon.ca
Acheson, AB

17200333R00150